Advances in Aortic Surgery

Edited by Takashi Murashita

Published in London, United Kingdom

Advances in Aortic Surgery
http://dx.doi.org/10.5772/intechopen.1009730
Edited by Takashi Murashita

Contributors
Chris White, Devin O'Brien, Ersin Ozer, Felipe Figueiró Teixeira, Hidayet Demir, Jacques Tomasi, Jakub Staromlynski, Jean-Philippe Verhoye, Mehmet Altuğ Tunçer, Mehrdad Sheikhvatan, Nilo César Barbosa Mandelli, Pedro Adolfo Mera Almonte, Pierre Escrig, Piotr Suwalski, Saurabh Gupta

First published in London, United Kingdom, 2026 by IntechOpen
IntechOpen is the global imprint of INTECHOPEN LIMITED, registered in England and Wales, registration number: 11086078, 167-169 Great Portland Street, London, W1W 5PF, United Kingdom

For EU product safety concerns: IN TECH d.o.o., Prolaz Marije Krucifikse Kozulić 3, 51000 Rijeka, Croatia, info@intechopen.com or visit our website at intechopen.com.

British Library Cataloguing-in-Publication Data
A catalogue record for this book is available from the British Library

Advances in Aortic Surgery
Edited by Takashi Murashita
p. cm.

This title is part of the Cardiology and Cardiovascular Medicine Book Series, Volume 16
Topic: Cardiovascular Surgery
Series Editor: Kaan Kırali
Topic Editor: Takashi Murashita

Print ISBN 978-1-83635-995-1
Online ISBN 978-1-83635-994-4
eBook (PDF) ISBN 978-1-83635-996-8
ISSN 3033-361X

IntechOpen Book Series

Cardiology and Cardiovascular Medicine

Volume 16

Aims and Scope of the Series

Today, since molecular science on structural causes of oncological pathologies and their molecular treatments are developing at an unbelievable rate, the primary medical cause of death in the twenty-first century will be cardiovascular disease. Neither pandemics that threaten all humanity nor deterioration in the ecosystem will be able to change this fact. Especially, this century seems poised to witness an incredible struggle against atherosclerotic disease, which develops in the arterial walls and results in narrowing and occlusion of the arterial lumen. In addition to this disease, there has been an increasing prevalence of heart rhythm problems, deterioration of heart valves due to aging, and heart failure. Serious vascular pathologies such as stenosis and occlusion, dissection and rupture, and aneurysmal enlargement are also major concerns. Medical and invasive treatment methods may work to save human lives, but they will never provide a real solution. All kinds of medical, technological, and genetic engineering developments obtained in these processes have not yet been sufficient to alleviate or eliminate cardiovascular disease. This book series, Cardiology and Cardiovascular Medicine, includes three topics. The first, Cardiovascular Diseases and Health, reviews important cardiovascular diseases and the developments in their prognosis. The second topic, Cardiovascular Electrophysiology, illuminates the abnormal functioning of the cardiac conduction system, which is caused by all heart pathologies and negatively affects prognosis. The third topic in this series, Cardiovascular Surgery, details treatment for cardiovascular pathologies and how to regulate normal physiological functions with percutaneous or extracorporeal interventions.

Meet the Series Editor

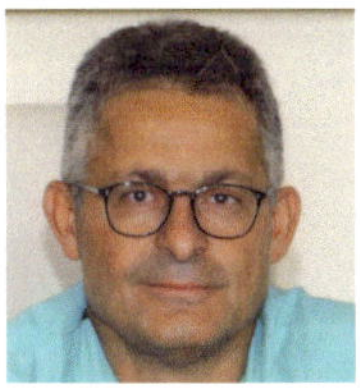

After completing his studies at the Medicine Faculty of Istanbul University in 1990, Prof. Kaan Kırali fulfilled his mandatory medical service and commenced his residency training at Koşuyolu Heart and Research Hospital in 1992. Following five years of assistant education, he pursued further training in England and the USA in 1998. Specializing in laparoscopic and minimally invasive cardiac surgery, he earned the titles of consultant cardiovascular surgeon in 1998, Assistant Professor in 1999, Associate Professor in 2002, and Chief in 2005 at the same hospital. Prof. Kırali also developed an interest in preventive medicine, obtaining an MSc in Public Health from Istanbul University in 2000. Over the past two decades, he has concentrated his scientific pursuits on cardiovascular repairs requiring specialized experience. With his expertise in coronary artery surgery, minimally invasive cardiac surgery, valve repair, and aortic root surgery, he has established new methods for awake coronary bypass revascularization, a new surgical approach for AVR during first and re-operations, aortic valve-sparing procedure, and radiofrequency ablation. Notably, he pioneered awake complete coronary artery bypass grafting (CABG) with bilateral internal mammary arteries (BIMA) and played a crucial role in advancing aortic root surgery with a new aortotomy incision, simplifying aortic valve interventions. Since the year 2000, Prof. Kırali has expanded his interests to heart transplantation, and in recent years, to left ventricular assist devices. He has served as the head of the transplantation department since 2015 and currently continues his work as the director of Koşuyolu High Specialization Education and Research Hospital in Istanbul, Turkey. In his prolific career, he has authored numerous papers in SCI journals, contributed to various book chapters, and served as an editor and reviewer for multiple academic journals. Additionally, he has edited several international books in the field of cardiovascular medicine.

Meet the Volume Editor

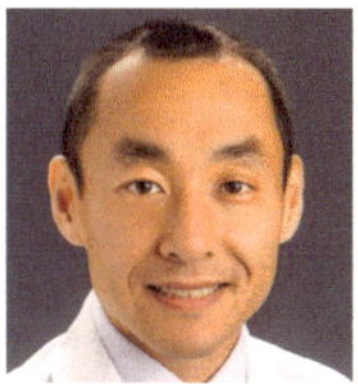

Takashi Murashita, MD, is an Assistant Professor at the Department of Surgery at Washington University in Saint Louis, MO, USA. Dr. Murashita received his MD from Kyoto University Medical School in Japan. His primary interest is cardiac surgery, and he is a member of the Society of Thoracic Surgery. He has published over 50 papers in peer-reviewed journals and 10 chapters in open-access books. He has been a member of the editorial boards of 2 medical journals and an ad hoc manuscript reviewer for over 15 medical journals.

Contents

Preface

The book, *Advances in Aortic Surgery*, is an excellent update for health care professionals caring for patients with complex aortic disease. Experts in their fields wrote the seven chapters in this book.

The first chapter discusses the optimal treatment for type A aortic dissection: hemiarch replacement versus total arch replacement. The authors provided excellent discussion points about the pros and cons of both procedures.

The second chapter discusses the long-term treatment strategy following repair of type A aortic dissection. The treatment for the remaining dissected aorta after type A dissection repair is always challenging. The authors provided the most up-to-date evidence on this topic.

The third chapter discusses the surgical treatment for aortic root disease. The authors described a variety of surgical techniques, including valve-sparing root replacement and Bentall operations.

The fourth chapter discusses a unique technique for thoracoabdominal aortic aneurysm. The surgery for a thoracoabdominal aortic aneurysm is associated with a high risk of complications. The authors described how to minimize the risk of the surgery.

The fifth chapter discusses the clinical and molecular aspects of abdominal aortic dissection, which is a rare clinical condition. The authors help us to understand the mechanisms of abdominal aortic dissection.

The sixth chapter discusses a hybrid approach for abdominal aortic aneurysm. The authors described the most recent evidence of a combination of open and endovascular treatments for complex abdominal aortic aneurysms.

The seventh chapter discusses current evidence of aortoiliac disease. The authors described a variety of surgical strategies for the management of aortoiliac disease.

Cardiovascular surgeons encounter a variety of complex aortic diseases. I believe this book will provide healthcare professionals with the most recent information on surgical interventions for complex aortic diseases.

Takashi Murashita, MD
Assistant Professor,
Division of Cardiothoracic Surgery,
Washington University,
iSaint Louis, MO, USA

Chapter 1

Hemiarch vs. Total Arch Replacement for Acute Type A Aortic Dissection

Devin O'Brien, Chris White and Saurabh Gupta

Abstract

Acute type A aortic dissection (ATAAD) is a catastrophic cardiovascular emergency, with mortality rising by 1–2% per hour if untreated. Emergent surgical intervention is the cornerstone of management, but the optimal extent of aortic arch repair is a matter of debate. The two principal strategies are hemiarch replacement (HAR) or total arch replacement (TAR). HAR involves resecting the ascending aorta into the proximal arch, reducing operative complexity, cardiopulmonary bypass, and circulatory arrest times, and is associated with lower early mortality and morbidity. However, HAR frequently leaves behind a residual dissected arch and descending aorta, leading to a persistent false lumen and aneurysmal degeneration, which often require future interventions. Conversely, TAR more definitively addresses arch pathology, promoting false lumen thrombosis and better distal aortic remodeling, with less reintervention required. However, this comes at the cost of higher perioperative risk, including increased mortality, renal failure, and neurologic complications in some series. This chapter will review the pathophysiology, classification, and surgical principles of ATAAD before critically appraising contemporary evidence comparing HAR and TAR. It will highlight the "gray zone" where either strategy may be justified. Emerging hybrid and stent-based adjuncts will be discussed. Ultimately, both strategies are valid, and the choice must be individualized based on patient anatomy, clinical stability, comorbidities, and institutional expertise.

Keywords: acute type A aortic dissection, hemiarch replacement, total arch replacement, extended arch repair, frozen elephant trunk, classic elephant trunk, surgical outcomes

1. Introduction

Acute aortic syndromes are classified into aortic dissections, intramural hematomas, and penetrating atherosclerotic ulcers [1]. Acute type A aortic dissection (ATAAD) is one of the most catastrophic cardiovascular emergencies in cardiac surgery [1–4]. If left untreated, mortality rates increase by 1–2% per hour during the first 24–48 hours; nearly half of these patients die within the first week of presentation without surgical intervention [1, 2, 4]. Despite improved diagnostic imaging modalities and new surgical techniques developed for treating ATAAD, mortality rates remain between 14 and 30% [3].

Surgery remains the definitive management strategy, but controversy persists regarding the extent of index repair. The two main strategies developed to manage an ATAAD are hemiarch replacement (HAR) or total arch replacement (TAR).

Hemiarch replacement involves resecting the ascending aorta, along with part of the proximal aortic arch. HAR reduces operative complexity and requires shorter cardiopulmonary bypass (CPB) and circulatory arrest times. In turn, this leads to lower perioperative mortality and morbidity [5, 6]. HAR can, however, leave a dissected distal aortic arch and descending thoracic aorta, often times with a persistent false lumen. This can increase the risk of late aneurysmal degeneration, reintervention requirements, or rupture [7, 8].

Total arch replacement involves complete resection and replacement of the aortic arch, and reimplantation of the head vessels. It is associated with increased operative complexity and perioperative risk, including – in some studies – higher rates of renal failure and early mortality [7]. However, it is especially advantageous when the primary intimal entry tear is located in the arch, and TAR is associated with improved rates of false lumen thrombosis and reduced long-term reintervention rates [6–9].

Both the 2022 ACC/AHA guidelines and the 2024 ESC guidelines recommend urgent surgery for all patients with ATAAD. Repair should entail at least an open distal anastomosis rather than a simple ascending aorta graft [1, 2]. However, neither guideline mandates TAR. The final decision regarding HAR or TAR must be individualized to better balance early operative safety and long-term durability, considering patient age, comorbidities, location of the primary tear, and institutional/surgeon expertise.

2. What is type A dissection?

2.1 Definition

Type A dissection is defined as an acute aortic dissection that involves the ascending aorta, regardless of whether it extends into the arch and descending thoracic aorta [1, 2]. Aortic dissection occurs in the event of an intimal tear, allowing blood to pass through the tear and into the medial layer, creating a newly formed false lumen. Antegrade or retrograde propagation of the dissection flap can lead to numerous complications, such as acute aortic regurgitation, tamponade, stroke, coronary artery compromise, and distal malperfusion [4]. The false lumen may remain patent, partially thrombosed, or fully thrombosed. The behavior of the false lumen can determine future complications, such as reentry tears, aneurysmal expansion, or aortic rupture [1, 2, 4].

2.2 Pathophysiology

ATAAD is associated with a combination of factors affecting wall stress and hemodynamic stressors, with chronic hypertension being the most common reason [2]. Inherited connective tissue disorders such as Marfan syndrome, Loeys–Dietz syndrome (LDS), and vascular Ehlers–Danlos syndrome (EDS) predispose the aorta to medial degeneration and intimal tearing at younger ages. Other risk factors include male sex, inflammatory aortitis, pregnancy, and abuse of stimulants like cocaine [1, 2].

2.3 Clinical presentation

Patients often present complaining of sudden, severe chest or back pain, typically described as tearing or ripping. Examination findings may include pulse deficits, blood pressure differentials, a new diastolic murmur, or clinical signs of tamponade. Neurologic deficits and ischemic end-organ injury are also common [1–7, 10].

2.4 Imaging

Computed tomography angiography (CTA) is the gold standard in acute diagnosis, with nearly 100% sensitivity and specificity. CTA not only portrays the intimal flap but also identifies the true and false lumen, as well as demonstrates the extent of the dissection and provides vital information about potential malperfusion. In unstable patients, transesophageal echocardiography may be considered. While magnetic resonance imaging provides excellent resolution, it is rarely practical in such an acute setting [1, 2, 4, 10].

2.5 Prognosis

Without surgery, ATAAD is generally fatal. International Registry of Acute Aortic Dissection (IRAD) data demonstrate that in-hospital mortality for untreated type A dissections exceeds 60% [1, 3, 4, 10]. Depending on factors such as the patient's stability, malperfusion, and surgeon/institutional experience, surgery can reduce in-hospital mortality to 15–25% [1, 2, 4].

3. Classification systems of type A dissection

3.1 Overview

Appropriate classification of acute aortic dissection is necessary for communication among the care team, allowing appropriate prognostication and therapeutic planning. Numerous classification systems have been proposed, with the Stanford and DeBakey classification systems still most widely used. However, more recent and nuanced frameworks, such as the Society for Vascular Surgery/Society of Thoracic Surgeons (SVS/STS) reporting standards, have been created to improve anatomical precision and surgical decision-making among aortic specialists [1, 2] (**Figure 1**).

3.2 Standford classification

The Stanford classification is based on whether the dissection involves the ascending aorta. Type A is described as any dissection involving the ascending aorta,

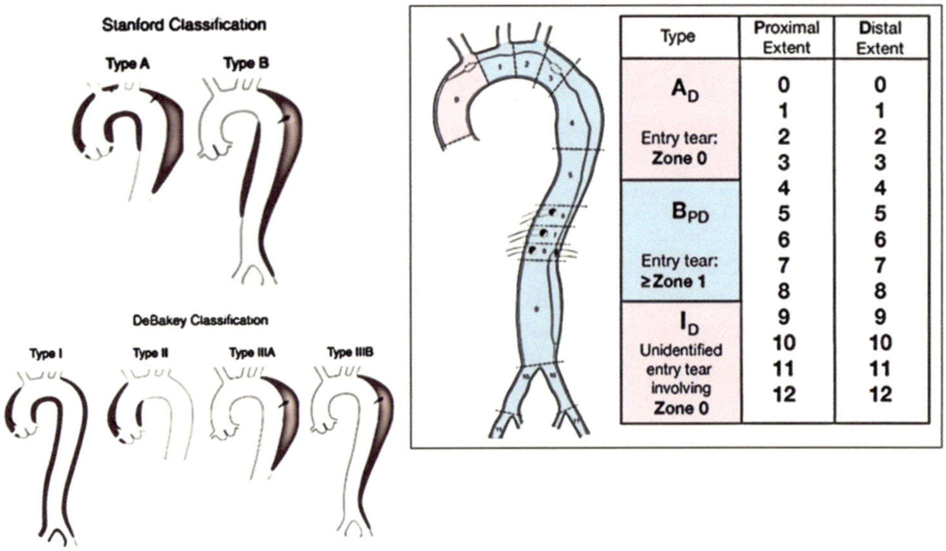

Figure 1.
Most common schemes used in describing type A dissections. Top left – Stanford classification, based on involvement of the ascending aorta or not. Bottom left – DeBakey classification, based on involvement of ascending aorta, with or without extension into distal aorta, as well as dissection of the descending aorta, with or without extension beyond the thoracic aorta. Top right – the latest SVS/STS classification, which aims to delineate the exact point of the entry tear (known or unknown), along with the proximal and distal extent. This is becoming more and more commonly utilized.

regardless of distal extension. Type B is described as being confined to the descending thoracic aorta, distal to the left subclavian artery. The simplicity of this classification has led to its prominent use in the medical community, with distinct management strategies: urgent surgery for type A and medical and/or endovascular therapy for the majority of type B [1, 2, 11, 12].

3.3 DeBakey classification

The DeBakey classification is based on the site of the intimal tear, as well as the extent of propagation. It is typically divided into three types:

- Type I – Originates in the ascending aorta and extends beyond the arch, often to the descending thoracic or abdominal aorta.
- Type II – Confined to the ascending aorta.
- Type III – Originates in the descending thoracic aorta, distal to the left subclavian artery. It is further subdivided into IIIa, which is confined to the thoracic aorta, and IIIb, which extends into the abdominal aorta.

While the DeBakey classification system provides more detail and is widely used in research and databases, it is less practical for emergency communications among medical professionals [1, 2, 11].

3.4 SVS/STS reporting standard

In 2010, the SVS/STS introduced a new segmental classification of the aorta to better identify entry and exit tear(s), along with their extent, in patients with aortic dissection. In 2020, they proposed a new classification system to define aortic dissection anatomy in more detail. This system defines dissections anatomically by the location of the intimal tear and the proximal and distal extent of the dissection [1, 2, 11, 12]. This classification system is increasingly popular in registries and trials, as well as among aortic specialists. It helps improve consistency across both surgical and endovascular studies.

3.5 TEM classification

Non-A, non-B dissections are characterized by dissections that are limited to the arch or retrograde dissections, which extend into the arch but not the ascending aorta [2, 13]. These types of dissections lead to a controversial surgical strategy, as many of these patients require TAR or hybrid approaches, since HAR risks leaving behind the entry tear.

While the description of non-A, non-B dissections has been around for some time, it has not been consistently used in research or the clinical setting. The TEM classification described in the 2024 ESC guidelines has reintroduced the concept of non-A, non-B dissections. This classification system characterizes dissections based on their type (A, B, non-A, non-B), entry tear location, and malperfusion [2, 13].

4. Evidence for surgery with type A dissection

4.1 Guideline-positioned principles

Internationally, there is guideline consensus that urgent surgery is required for most ATAAD. In addition, operative repair should include – at minimum – an open distal anastomosis, rather than a supracoronary graft, given that open distal repair improves resection of the intimal tear and promotes distal remodeling [1, 2, 14]. While guidelines do not recommend TAR for all ATAAD patients, they recommend tailoring the extent of arch work based on the patient's anatomy (location of tear or aneurysm) and age, as well as any evidence of concomitant descending thoracic aortic aneurysm, distal malperfusion, or connective tissue disorders.

4.2 Contemporary evidence: Hemiarch vs. TAR

The most current comparative analysis of hemiarch vs. total arch repair in ATAAD is a meta-analysis by Hage et al. (2024). They analyzed 22 comparative studies, including 6,526 patients. They reported:

- 30-day/early mortality: higher with TAR (OR 1.79, 95% CI 1.29–2.49).
- Renal failure requiring dialysis: higher with TAR (OR 1.34, 95% CI 1.02–1.76).
- Stroke: potentially higher with TAR (OR 1.49, 95% CI 0.93–2.39).

- Late aortic reoperations: potentially fewer with TAR (HR 0.53; 95% CI 0.18–1.59).

- Subgroup analysis: It is important to note that a potential increase in long-term mortality with TAR was observed mostly in studies where the prevalence of malperfusion was 10% higher in patients undergoing TAR compared to the patients undergoing HAR. This suggests patient selection influenced the crude comparisons.

HAR generally has lower perioperative risk, while TAR may reduce late distal events/reintervention [5–9]. These trade-offs are in keeping with the guidelines' emphasis on individualized strategies for ATAAD repair [1, 2, 14].

4.3 Early outcomes

Despite continued advances, surgical mortality for ATAAD remains substantial. However, in-hospital mortality has decreased in more recent reports because of advancements in surgical strategies and improvements in cerebral protection strategies [4].

No matter, literature continues to report greater perioperative risk with TAR when compared to HAR. Kim et al. (2011) found significantly greater adjusted mortality in TAR patients (HR 2.38), along with a higher risk of permanent neurologic injury (HR 3.25). These findings are supported by the Hage et al. (2024) meta-analysis, which showed higher 30-day mortality and renal failure with TAR, as well as a trend toward higher stroke rates. Due to the increased risks with TAR, the Canadian Thoracic Aortic Collaborative (CTAC) highlights that unstable patients may benefit from a simpler operation and recommends HAR. Extended repairs are typically reasonable when the primary intimal tear is in the distal arch or descending aorta, in young patients or in patients with known connective tissue disorders, and when there is evidence of a dilated arch or descending thoracic aorta [14].

While neurological complications continue to be a concern, the difference between HAR and TAR is becoming less apparent. Although some studies may still report statistically significant new neurologic injuries with TAR [5], a few others show no statistically significant difference between either strategy [7, 15]. This improvement may be due to the adoption of strategies like bilateral antegrade cerebral perfusion. While renal failure is naturally expected to be higher in TAR due to longer CPB and circulatory arrest times, studies also show conflicting results here too [7, 15].

4.4 Late outcomes

HAR offers lower early mortality, but its limitation lies in the persistent false lumen in the distal aorta. IRAD data demonstrate that continued perfusion of the false lumen is linked to distal aortic enlargement and further adverse late outcomes [4, 7, 8]. Multiple surgical series and studies have confirmed this; patients who underwent HAR often experienced distal aortic growth and eventually required further intervention [14]. Rylski et al. (2017) reinforced this concept by analyzing ATAAD patients with residual dissection. An average growth rate of 1.5 mm per year was observed, as well as approximately 15% of patients requiring late reintervention.

These findings support concerns about leaving the arch and descending thoracic aorta dissected and predisposing patients to long-term aneurysmal degeneration.

In contrast, TAR is linked to improved distal remodeling and reduced need for secondary procedures, especially when combined with adjuncts such as the frozen elephant trunk (FET). The International E-vita Registry shows that FET led to immediate complete false lumen thrombosis in 86% of patients, increasing to 94% at the latest follow-up, while maintaining acceptable mortality rates [9]. The Hage et al. (2024) meta-analysis further solidifies this, showing a trend toward fewer late reoperations and improved distal remodeling with TAR. However, despite these positive benefits, there was no significant long-term survival advantage, signifying that the benefits of TAR could be more structural than survival-related.

Based on the available literature, HAR provides superior early outcomes, while TAR offers improved distal remodeling and fewer reinterventions, especially in anatomically favorable candidates or those with arch tears. Despite these outcomes, a survival advantage is not consistently demonstrated, highlighting the importance of individualized decision-making and careful follow-up for all ATAAD patients.

5. The gray zone

Current guidelines and registry data provide clear direction for unstable patients and those with well-defined arch involvement; however, a proportion of ATAAD patients fall into a "gray zone" where both HAR and TAR could be justified. The doubt is rooted in balancing immediate operative risk with the long-term sequelae of leaving behind dissected aortic tissue. Aside from the patient profile, another important aspect of choosing appropriately lies in the surgeon's and institutional experience.

Hemodynamically stable patients with an ambiguous primary entry tear that is close to, but not definitively within the arch often fit into this gray zone. While HAR is a shorter and safer operation in patients who are already at high baseline mortality risk, registries show that if there is true arch pathology, a more extensive approach using TAR with FET results in favorable remodeling and lower rates of reintervention [9]. Depending on preoperative imaging and intra-operative inspection, either strategy could be defended.

Another group for which both strategies could be argued are young patients without major comorbidities. Limiting the initial operation to HAR may increase survival from the acute event in unstable or high-risk cases, but younger patients will likely face decades of life expectancy following their initial operation, which may necessitate a more aggressive initial approach [14]. In younger patients, surgeons should likely consider survival vs. durability, while also balancing the patient's initial presentation and clinical status. Another consideration for young patients regarding which procedure to perform is the amount of follow-up imaging they will need, given the amount of radiation they will be exposed to over the years. On the opposite spectrum, elderly or frail patients may benefit from shorter CPB and circulatory arrest times to minimize neurological and renal insult, even if they present with a tear in the arch.

Connective tissue disorder patients, such as those with Marfan syndrome, LDS, or vascular EDS, also become complex to manage. Given their severe tissue fragility, one could argue for performing the lower complexity HAR procedure, while others could argue that late dilation of the distal aorta is more likely, and a more definitive arch management should be undertaken. These patients also require consideration of what secondary procedures they will need based on the choice of the primary operation, as endovascular repairs are less favorable in connective tissue disorder patients.

Major international guidelines from Canada, the United States of America, and Europe reflect the ambiguity of HAR vs. TAR by endorsing hemiarch as a baseline operative strategy but allowing for extensive repair in experienced centers with experienced surgeons, and when the patient population and anatomy suggest potential for long-term benefit [1, 2, 14].

6. Options to manage the aortic arch in acute type A dissection

6.1 Hemiarch replacement

The standard approach for ATAAD patients with tears confined to the ascending aorta is a HAR. This involves resection of the ascending aorta up to the origin of the innominate artery, with a bevel into the lesser curvature of the arch. The distal end is anastomosed open, with deep hypothermic circulatory arrest, with or without cerebral perfusion (depending on the patient's acuity) [13, 14]. Some surgeons may choose to perform HAR for ATAAD under moderate hypothermic circulatory arrest, but we recommend lower temperatures in case more extensive work is required.

6.2 Total arch replacement

When the intimal tear extends into the arch or when the arch is dilated, TAR is the appropriate option. TAR is generally done with branched grafts – the Kazui four-branched or Spielvogel Y-graft, for example – to reimplant the supra-aortic vessels. This procedure is generally reserved for experienced surgeons and patients with arch tears, connective tissue disease, malperfusion, and younger patients [13, 14].

6.3 Hybrid arch approaches

Hybrid arch approaches are becoming increasingly popular as an added tool for experienced aortic endovascular surgeons. This approach combines the surgical rerouting of the arch vessels with an endovascular stent graft deployed into the descending aorta. The major benefit of this approach is that it can create a stable proximal landing zone for future endovascular stenting. Given its relatively recent emergence, there is limited long-term data [13, 14].

6.4 Extended arch approaches

Currently, there are three major categories of extended arch approaches: classic elephant trunk (CET), FET, and the Ascyrus Medical Dissection Stent (AMDS). The CET involves sewing a free-floating Dacron graft extension – known as the elephant trunk – into the proximal descending thoracic aorta during a TAR. FET combines TAR with the antegrade deployment of a stented graft into the descending thoracic aorta during the same operation.

Advantages of CET include a simplified distal aortic arch anastomosis, facilitation of future thoracoabdominal aortic interventions (open or endovascular), and lower expense. However, given that a staged procedure is needed, there is a high mortality rate in the interval between staged procedures, and it does not promote distal aortic remodeling by itself [16] (**Figure 2**).

FET, conversely, allows for single-stage treatment, facilitates future endovascular thoracoabdominal aortic interventions, and reduces the risk of additional distal aortic surgery. With FET, there is also no stent migration since the proximal aspect is sewn surgically, limited to no risk of type 1a endoleak, and it reduces the risk of ongoing malperfusion and promotes distal aortic remodeling [16]. Some literature goes as far as to say TAR with FET may become a new "standard" therapy [17]. The standard options for FET are either the "E-Vita Open Neo" stent graft system or the "Terumo Thoraflex" (**Figure 2**).

Unfortunately, FET is associated with an increased incidence of thromboembolic complications, with one study finding a rate of 12%, occurring more commonly with the 150 mm stent graft [18]. A multicenter national registry found that there was no difference in stroke or in-hospital mortality between HAR and extended arch repair strategies [19]. The CTAC database found no difference in stroke between CET and FET, reporting higher mortality with CET (13%) vs. FET (9%) and a higher risk of spinal cord injury with FET compared to CET (odds ratio: 2.20; 95% CI: 1.10–4.37) [20].

A more recent development in extended arch approaches is the AMDS (**Figure 2**), which was designed as an adjunct to the hemiarch repair. It is not only useful for aortic-trained surgeons but also beneficial for cardiac surgeons with limited aortic experience who are performing ATAAD repairs. This is an uncovered antegrade stent that is deployed into the arch during circulatory arrest and extends into the

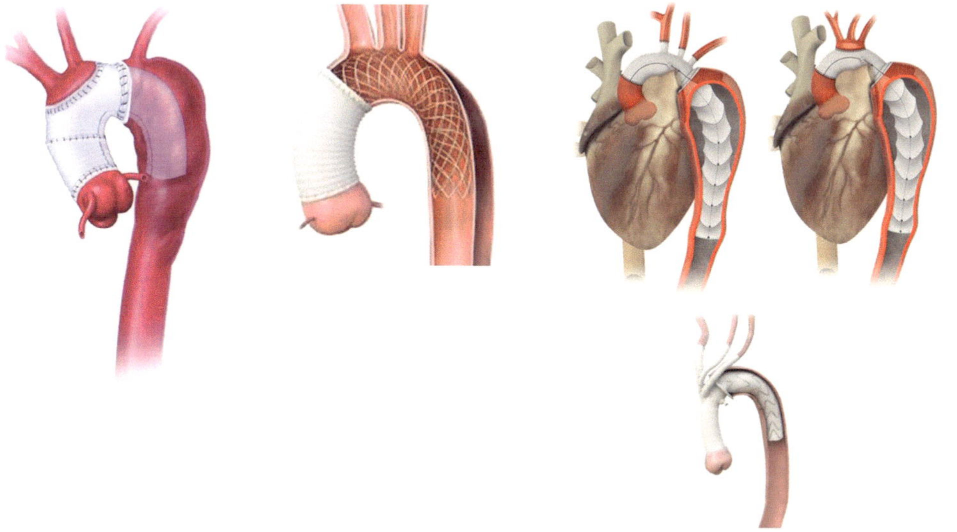

Figure 2.
Various ways to manage the arch. Top left – classic elephant trunk. Top center – AMDS stent, which allows for expansion of the true lumen without extensive arch surgery. Top right – FET with the Terumo Thoraflex. Bottom right – FET with the E-vita graft.

proximal descending aorta. It promotes true lumen expansion and false lumen thrombosis.

7. Conclusion

ATAAD continues to represent one of the most formidable challenges in cardiovascular surgery, carrying high rates of morbidity and mortality despite improvements in diagnostic imaging, surgical strategy, and perioperative care. The essential principle is that all operable patients require urgent surgical repair, with an open distal anastomosis extending into the proximal arch.

Debate remains around the choice between HAR and TAR. HAR offers reduced operative complexity, shorter circulatory arrest and CPB times, and lower perioperative mortality but often leaves residual dissected aorta that predisposes patients to late aneurysmal degeneration and reintervention. TAR, while more technically demanding and associated with higher perioperative complications, promotes distal aortic remodeling, reduces the risk of, and from, a persistent false lumen, and lowers the risk of later reinterventions, particularly when combined with FET or a CET.

Registry data, meta-analyses, and guideline recommendations converge on the importance of tailoring the extent of arch repair to individual patient factors: age, comorbidities, connective tissue disorders, tear location, and stability at presentation, along with institutional and surgeon expertise. Patients in the "gray zone," including those with ambiguous tear location, younger patients with long life expectancy, and those with connective tissue disease, illustrate the nuanced decision-making required to balance early safety with long-term durability.

Emerging strategies, such as hybrid arch approaches, FET, and the AMDS, continue to expand the surgical toolkit. These options reflect an evolution toward integrating open and endovascular techniques, with the aim of minimizing operative risk while maximizing long-term aortic stability.

Ultimately, there is no one-size-fits-all solution. HAR remains the baseline operation for many centers, while TAR and extended arch strategies offer improved durability in carefully selected patients. Continued international collaboration, long-term registry data, and randomized studies will be essential to refine these strategies further. This is currently being examined in the ARCH registry [21]. Furthermore, the Canadian-led TITAN:HEADSTART (hemiarch vs. extended arch in type 1 aortic dissection) should also provide us with extremely important insights into the management of ATAAD patients. This is a prospective, open-label, non-blinded, multicenter, randomized controlled trial that aims to compare HAR with extended arch repair (TAR or HAR with AMDS) for ATAAD. The current estimated enrollment aim is for 50 patients [22].

For now, it is clear that early diagnosis, urgent operative management, and individualized surgical planning are the cornerstones of improving outcomes in ATAAD.

Conflicts of Interest

The authors declare no conflict of interest.

Author details

Devin O'Brien[1], Chris White[2] and Saurabh Gupta[2*]

1 University of Alberta, Mazankowski Alberta Heart Institute, Division of Cardiac Surgery, Edmonton, Canada

2 Dalhousie University, New Brunswick Heart Centre, Division of Cardiac Surgery, Saint John, Canada

*Address all correspondence to: soreabgupta@gmail.com

References

[1] Isselbacher EM, Preventza O, Black 3rd JH, Augoustides JG, Beck AW, Bolen MA, Braverman AC, Bray BE, Brown-Zimmerman MM, Chen EP, Collins TJ, De Anda AJ, Fanola CL, Girardi LN, Hicks CW, Hui DS, Jones WS, Kalahasti V, Kim KM, Milewicz DM, Oderich GS, Ogbechie L, Promes SB, Ross EG, Schermerhorn ML, Times SS, Tseng EE, Wang GJ, Woo YJ. ACC/AHA guideline for the diagnosis and management of aortic disease: A report of the American Heart Association/American College of Cardiology Joint Committee on Clinical Practice Guidelines. Circulation. 2022;**146**(24):e334–e482. DOI: 10.1161/CIR.0000000000001106

[2] Mazzolai L, Teixido-Tura G, Lanzi S, Boc V, Bossone E, Brodmann M, Bura-Rivière A, De Backer J, Deglise S, Della Corte A, Heiss C, Kałużna-Oleksy M, Kurpas D, McEniery CM, Mirault T, Pasquet AA, Pitcher A, Schaubroeck HAI, Schlager O, Sirnes PA, Sprynger MG, Stabile E, Steinbach F, Thielmann M, van Kimmenade RRJ, Venermo M, Rodriguez-Palomares JF; ESC Scientific Document Group. ESC Guidelines for the management of peripheral arterial and aortic diseases. European Heart Journal. 2024;**45**(36):3538–3700. DOI: 10.1093/eurheartj/ehae179

[3] Pape LA, Tsai TT, Isselbacher EM, Oh JK, O'Gara PT, Evangelista A, Fattori R, Meinhardt G, Trimarchi S, Bossone E, Suzuki T, Cooper JV, Froehlich JB, Nienaber CA, Eagle KA. International Registry of Acute Aortic Dissection (IRAD) investigators. aortic diameter ≥5.5 cm is not a good predictor of type A aortic dissection: Observations from the International Registry of Acute Aortic Dissection (IRAD). Circulation. 2007;**116** (10):1120–1127. DOI: 10.1161/CIRCULATIONAHA.107.702720

[4] Pape LA, Awais M, Woznicki EM, Suzuki T, Trimarchi S, Evangelista A, Myrmel T, Larsen M, Harris KM, Greason K, Di Eusanio M, Bossone E, Montgomery DG, Eagle KA, Nienaber CA, Isselbacher EM, O'Gara P. Presentation, diagnosis, and outcomes of acute aortic dissection: 17-year trends from the International Registry of Acute Aortic Dissection. Journal of the American College of Cardiology. 2015;**66**(4):350–358. DOI: 10.1016/j.jacc.2015.05.029

[5] Kim JB, Chung CH, Moon DH, Ha GJ, Lee TY, Jung SH, Choo SJ, Lee JW. Total arch repair versus hemiarch repair in the management of acute DeBakey type I aortic dissection. European Journal of Cardio-thoracic Surgery : Official Journal of the European Association for Cardio-thoracic Surgery. 2011;**40**(4): 881–889. DOI: 10.1016/j.ejcts.2010.12.035

[6] Li B, Ma WG, Liu YM, Sun LZ. Is extended arch replacement justified for acute type A aortic dissection? Interactive CardioVascular and Thoracic Surgery. 2015;**20**(1):120–127. DOI: 10.1093/icvts/ivu323

[7] Hage F, Atarere J, Anteby R, Hage A, Malik MI, Boodhwani M, Ouzounian M, Chu MWA. Total arch vs hemiarch repair in acute type A aortic dissection: Systematic review and meta-analysis of comparative studies. CJC Open. 2024;**6** (4):1075–1086. DOI: 10.1016/j.cjco.2024.04.012

[8] Rylski B, Hahn N, Beyersdorf F, Kondov S, Wolkewitz M, Blanke P, Plonek T, Czerny M, Siepe M. Fate of the dissected aortic arch after ascending replacement in type A aortic dissection. European Journal of Cardio-Thoracic Surgery. 2017;**51**(6):1127–1134. DOI: 10.1093/ejcts/ezx062

[9] Tsagakis K, Pacini D, Di Bartolomeo R, Gorlitzer M, Weiss G, Grabenwoger M, Mestres CA, Benedik J, Cerny S, Jakob H. Multicenter early experience with extended aortic repair in acute aortic dissection: Is simultaneous descending stent grafting justified? the Journal of Thoracic and Cardiovascular Surgery. 2010;**140** (6 Suppl):S116–S120. DOI: 10.1016/j.jtcvs.2010.07.066

[10] Hagan PG, Nienaber CA, Isselbacher EM, et al. The International Registry of Acute Aortic Dissection (IRAD): New insights into an old disease. JAMA. 2000;**283**(7):897–903. DOI: 10.1001/jama.283.7.897

[11] Hiratzka LF, Bakris GL, Beckman JA, Bersin RM, Carr VF, DE Jr C, Eagle KA, Hermann LK, Isselbacher EM, Kazerooni EA, Kouchoukos NT, Lytle BW, Milewicz DM, Reich DL, Sen S, Shinn JA, Svensson LG, Williams DM. 2010 ACCF/AHA/AATS/ACR/ASA/SCA/SCAI/SIR/STS/SVM guidelines for the diagnosis and management of patients with thoracic aortic disease: a report of the American College of Cardiology Foundation/American Heart Association Task Force on Practice Guidelines, American Association for Thoracic Surgery, American College of Radiology, American Stroke Association, Society of Cardiovascular Anesthesiologists, Society for Cardiovascular Angiography and Interventions, Society of Interventional Radiology, Society of Thoracic Surgeons, and Society for Vascular Medicine. Circulation. 2010;**121**(13): e266–e369. DOI: 10.1161/CIR.0b013e3181d4739e

[12] Lombardi JV, Hughes GC, Appoo JJ, Bavaria JE, Beck AW, Cambria RP, Charlton-Ouw K, Eslami MH, Kim KM, Leshnower BG, Maldonado T, Reece TB, Wang GJ. Society for Vascular Surgery (SVS) and Society of Thoracic Surgeons (STS). Society for Vascular Surgery (SVS) and Society of Thoracic Surgeons (STS) reporting standards for type B aortic dissections. Journal of Vascular Surgery. 2020;**71**(3):723–747. DOI: 10.1016/j.jvs.2019.11.013

[13] Czerny M, Schmidli J, Adler S, van den Berg JC, Bertoglio L, Carrel T, Chiesa R, Clough RE, Eberle B, Etz C, Grabenwöger M, Haulon S, Jakob H, Kari FA, Mestres CA, Pacini D, Resch T, Rylski B, Schoenhoff F, Shrestha M, von Tengg-kobligk H, Tsagakis K, Wyss TR; EACTS/ESVS Scientific Document Group. Current options and recommendations for the treatment of thoracic aortic pathologies involving the aortic arch: An expert consensus document of the European Association for Cardio-Thoracic Surgery (EACTS) and the European Society for Vascular Surgery (ESVS). European Journal of Vascular and Endovascular Surgery : the Official Journal of the European Society for Vascular Surgery. 2019;**57**(2): 165–198. DOI: 10.1016/j.ejvs.2018.09.016

[14] El-Hamamsy I, Ouzounian M, Demers P, McClure S, Hassan A, Dagenais F, Chu MWA, Pozeg Z, Bozinovski J, Peterson MD, Boodhwani M, McArthur RGG, Appoo JJ. Canadian Thoracic Aortic Collaborative (CTAC). State-of-the-art

surgical management of acute type A aortic dissection. The Canadian Journal of Cardiology. 2016;**32**(1): 100–109. DOI: 10.1016/j.cjca.2015.07.736

[15] Zhang H, Lang X, Lu F, Song Z, Wang J, Han L, Xu Z. Acute type A dissection without intimal tear in arch: Proximal or extensive repair? the Journal of Thoracic and Cardiovascular Surgery. 2014;**147**(4):1251–1255. DOI: 10.1016/j.jtcvs.2013.04.029

[16] Di Bartolomeo R, Murana G, Di Marco L, Pantaleo A, Alfonsi J, Leone A, Pacini D. Frozen versus conventional elephant trunk technique: Application in clinical practice. European Journal of Cardio-Thoracic Surgery. 2017;**51**(Suppl 1):i25–i33. DOI: 10.1093/ejcts/ezw335

[17] Sun L, Qi R, Zhu J, Liu Y, Zheng J. Total arch replacement combined with stented elephant trunk implantation: A new "standard" therapy for type A dissection involving repair of the aortic arch? Circulation. 2011;**123** (9):971–978. DOI: 10.1161/CIRCULATIONAHA.110.015081

[18] Ibrahim M, Chung JC, Ascaso M, et al. In-hospital thromboembolic complications after frozen elephant trunk aortic arch repair. The Journal of Thoracic and Cardiovascular Surgery. 2024;**167**(4):1217–1226. DOI: 10.1016/j.jtcvs.2022.08.005

[19] Elbatarny M, Stevens LM, Dagenais F, et al. Hemiarch versus extended arch repair for acute type A dissection: Results from a multicenter national registry. The Journal of Thoracic and Cardiovascular Surgery. 2024;**167**(3):935–943.e5. DOI: 10.1016/j.jtcvs.2023.04.012

[20] Hage A, Hage F, Dagenais F, et al. Frozen elephant trunk for aortic arch reconstruction is associated with reduced mortality as compared to conventional techniques. Seminars in Thoracic and Cardiovascular Surgery. 2022;**34**(2):386–392. DOI: 10.1053/j.semtcvs.2021.03.049

[21] Nappi F, Schoell T, Singh SSA, et al. Aortic arch registry of type A aortic dissection (AoArch) - rationale, design and definition criteria. Journal of Cardiothoracic Surgery. 2024;**19**(1):514. DOI: 10.1186/s13019-024-03002-4

[22] Hemiarch Vs Extended Type 1 Aortic Dissection (HEADSTART). NCT 03885635. University of Ottawa Heart Institute Research Corporation. https://clinicaltrials.gov/study/NCT03885635 [Accessed: October-18]

Chapter 2

Management of Chronic Aortic Dissections After Type A: How and When to Reintervene

Jacques Tomasi, Pierre Escrig and Jean-Philippe Verhoye

Abstract

Acute Stanford type A aortic dissection is a surgical emergency with increasing survival due to advances in operative techniques. However, the majority of patients are left with a chronically dissected distal aorta – referred to as residual dissection after type A repair – which carries a substantial long-term risk of aneurysmal degeneration, rupture, and malperfusion. Up to 30–40% of survivors may require secondary interventions within two decades. Contemporary guidelines (ACC/AHA 2022, ESC 2024, EACTS/STS 2024) recommend lifelong surveillance, strict blood pressure control, and timely elective reintervention when defined thresholds are reached. Indications include aneurysm diameter ≥5.0–5.5 cm, rapid growth, new symptoms, or branch vessel malperfusion. Therapeutic options encompass open surgical reintervention, thoracic endovascular aortic repair (TEVAR), and hybrid approaches such as frozen elephant trunk, with choice tailored to anatomy, patient risk profile, and institutional expertise. Open surgery remains the gold standard in young and connective tissue disorder patients, offering durable exclusion of the false lumen, while TEVAR provides a less invasive alternative promoting favorable remodeling in selected anatomies. Hybrid strategies expand applicability in complex arch or thoracoabdominal disease. Outcomes have improved significantly in high-volume centers, with elective mortality in single digits and long-term survival comparable to nonreintervened patients. A multidisciplinary aortic team and proactive imaging-guided management are essential to optimize long-term outcomes for this challenging patient population.

Keywords: type A aortic dissection, chronic dissection, residual dissection, reintervention, aortic aneurysm, open surgery, thoracic endovascular aortic repair (TEVAR), frozen elephant trunk, hybrid aortic repair, aortic surgery outcomes

1. Introduction

Acute Stanford type A aortic dissection is a life-threatening emergency that requires prompt surgical repair of the ascending aorta (and often the proximal arch) to prevent rupture or cardiac tamponade [1–5]. Thanks to improved surgical techniques, many patients survive the acute repair; however, a majority are left with a residual dissection in the distal aorta beyond the surgical graft. In fact, a patent false lumen in the descending aorta is the most common scenario among survivors of type A dissection repair (observed in ~43–77% of cases) [6]. This chronically dissected residual aorta carries a substantial risk of progressive dilation (aneurysm formation), the need for reintervention, and late mortality [7]. Close lifelong surveillance of the entire aorta is therefore essential to improve long-term outcomes [8]. Importantly, a significant proportion of patients will ultimately require a secondary intervention on the distal aorta: studies report that roughly 10–20% of patients need aortic reintervention within 5–10 years after an acute type A dissection repair, and some series document rates as high as 30–40% with longer follow-up [9]. These reinterventions intend to prevent late catastrophic complications (such as aneurysm rupture or malperfusion) but pose significant challenges, often involving complex arch or thoracoabdominal procedures [6, 10–38].

Despite the frequency of chronic dissections after type A repair, dedicated management guidelines have only recently emerged. The 2022 ACC/AHA, 2024 ESC, and 2024 EACTS/STS guidelines now provide specific criteria for surveillance and reintervention in patients with chronic residual dissection, emphasizing lifelong imaging, intervention at defined diameter thresholds, and individualized management for heritable aortopathies [6–8]. The term "residual dissection after type A repair" has been introduced to describe the chronically dissected aortic segments distal to the surgical graft [10, 11]. This chapter will review the approach to these chronic residual dissections, focusing on when reintervention is indicated and how to choose the optimal therapy. Key considerations include patient surveillance, indications for reintervention (e.g., aneurysm size, growth rate, or symptoms), and the available treatment modalities – ranging from continued medical management to open surgical reoperations, endovascular repair, or hybrid approaches. The goal is to prevent adverse events like rupture while minimizing procedure-related risks, all tailored by a multidisciplinary aortic team on a case-by-case basis [7, 12, 39–49].

2. Surveillance and medical management after type A dissection

Long-term surveillance is critical for patients with a residual aortic dissection after type A repair. Immediately after the acute operation, patients should be maintained on rigorous medical therapy to control blood pressure and reduce shear stress on the aortic wall. Beta-blockers (and other antihypertensives) are commonly used to target a blood pressure around 120/80 mmHg or lower (if tolerated), as strict blood pressure control has been associated with slower aortic expansion. In patients with connective tissue disorders (e.g., Marfan syndrome), angiotensin receptor blockers are often added for their potential protective effect on the aorta. Although specific pharmacologic trials in chronic dissection are lacking, these medical measures are extrapolated from acute dissection management and aneurysm guidelines and are considered standard care to prevent false lumen pressurization and growth [6–9].

Imaging follow-up protocol: After the initial repair, a baseline high-quality scan (typically CT angiography) is obtained before discharge or within the first month to document the postsurgical aortic anatomy. Thereafter, current expert recommendations are to perform imaging at 6 months, at 12 months, and annually thereafter if the aorta remains stable [**Figure 1**] [13]. Patients managed

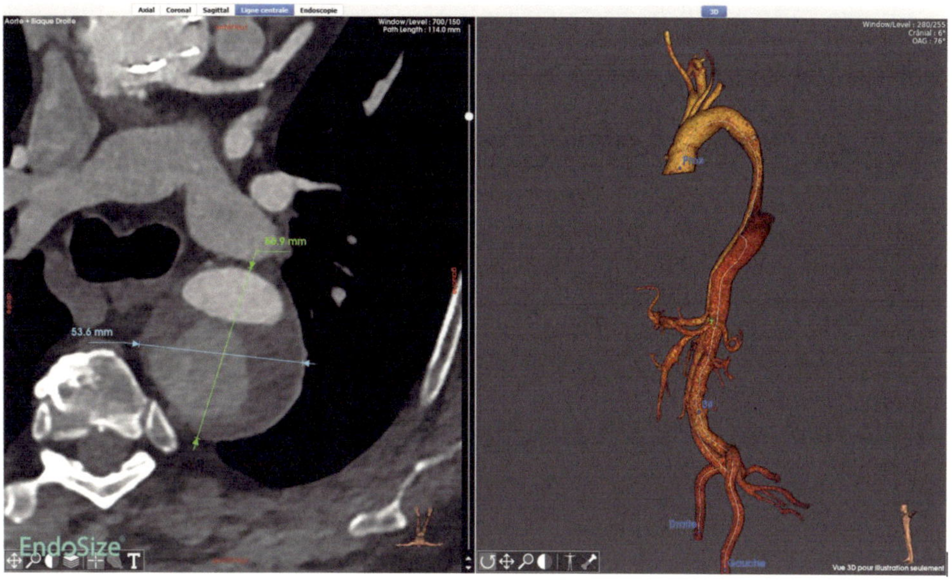

Figure 1.
Chronic aortic dissection at four years of follow-up. On the left, a CT scan shows the true lumen and a partially thrombosed false channel with a descending aortic dilatation. On the, a 3D reconstruction highlights the compression of the true lumen and the extension of the false channel.

nonoperatively for distal dissection (or those with endografts) may be imaged even more frequently in the first year (e.g., at 3 months) [14]. Surveillance imaging should cover the entire aorta, from the arch to the iliac arteries, since any segment of the residual dissection can evolve over time [15]. Over the long term, if the aorta shows no significant changes after a few years, the interval can be cautiously extended (e.g., to every 2–3 years), but lifelong periodic imaging is mandatory. Whenever possible, the same imaging modality and measurement technique should be used each time to ensure consistent comparisons [16]. CT angiography is the gold standard for anatomic detail and planning; however, in younger patients or those requiring very long-term surveillance, MR angiography can be considered to minimize cumulative radiation. Transthoracic or transesophageal echocardiography is useful for evaluating the proximal aortic root and valve, but it cannot reliably track the distal arch or descending aorta – thus, echocardiography is an adjunct to CT/MR rather than a replacement in this context [1].

During follow-up, clinicians must be vigilant for signs of aortic expansion or late complications. Aneurysm formation is very common in chronic postdissection aortas; studies have found aneurysmal degeneration in up to 49% of patients who had a residual dissection after type A repair (by comparison, about one-third of chronic type B dissections managed medically will develop aneurysms over time [2]). The typical remodeling pattern in residual type A dissection is slow expansion of the dissected descending thoracic aorta over years, due to pressurization of the false lumen. Any increase in aortic diameter should be noted; an expansion rate >2–3 mm per year is concerning, and rapid growth of >10 mm/year is generally considered an indication for intervention in chronic dissection [3]. The presence of persistent perfusion of the false lumen, especially with multiple reentry tears, strongly predicts progressive enlargement. Some imaging features associated with faster growth include a large false lumen (especially if it equals or exceeds the true lumen in size), continued patency of the false channel (paradoxically, partial thrombosis may be even more ominous than full thrombosis in terms of growth rate), and a large initial postoperative diameter (e.g., a descending aorta >40 mm early after surgery) [17].

In addition to imaging, clinical follow-up is important. Patients should be educated about symptoms that could herald a complication: New chest, back, or abdominal pain (which could indicate rapid expansion or a new tear) should prompt immediate evaluation [18]. Likewise, any signs of branch-vessel malperfusion – such as renal dysfunction, abdominal pain after meals (mesenteric ischemia), or limb ischemia – in a patient with known chronic dissection should raise concern for dynamic obstruction or progression of the dissection flap, warranting urgent imaging [19]. Though rare in the chronic phase, late complications like frank aortic rupture can occur (estimated in 3–18% of chronic dissections) and typically present with acute pain and hemodynamic collapse [20]. Thus, maintaining a high index of suspicion during long-term care is crucial.

Risk factor stratification: Recent research has identified several factors that predict which patients are most likely to require reintervention due to aneurysmal degeneration after a type A dissection repair. These include younger patient age (younger survivors have longer exposure time and often more aggressive disease) and male sex [39]. Certain aortic characteristics also confer higher risk: For example, a bicuspid aortic valve or an underlying connective tissue disorder (Marfan, Loeys-Dietz, etc.) are known to predispose to faster aortic enlargement and thus may justify closer monitoring or earlier elective intervention [50]. Anatomically, as noted, an initial descending aorta diameter >40 mm, a persistently patent false lumen, and either an unresected primary intimal tear or additional distal reentry tears all facilitate ongoing pressurization of the false channel [40]. The concept of the "distal anastomosis new entry" (DANE) has also been described: If the surgical repair's distal suture line is in dissected aorta (e.g., a limited ascending replacement), it can create a new tear or entry point at that junction, which keeps the false lumen open and prone to expansion [51]. Furthermore, the ratio of true lumen to false lumen area on early follow-up scans can be prognostic – for instance, a TL/FL area ratio <1 (i.e., false lumen larger than true lumen) within the first three months postop is associated with later aneurysm formation [52]. All these factors help identify patients who might benefit from closer surveillance intervals or even preemptive intervention. Indeed, in high-risk situations (such as a rapidly expanding false lumen or a young Marfan patient with a 45–50 mm dissected aorta), some centers advocate early elective stent-graft or surgical treatment before the standard size threshold is reached [53]. This proactive strategy aims to induce false lumen thrombosis and stabilize the aorta, potentially improving long-term survival [21]. However, given the nontrivial risks of intervention, such an approach must be balanced against procedural risk – underscoring the need for multidisciplinary case-by-case deliberation in an expert Aortic Center [54, 55].

In summary, meticulous medical management and surveillance are the foundation of managing chronic residual dissections. By optimizing medical therapy and tracking aortic changes over time, clinicians can determine the ideal timing of reintervention – intervening early enough to prevent rupture or malperfusion, but not so early as to subject the patient to unnecessary risk. In the sections below, we discuss the specific indications for reintervention and the therapeutic options available [6–8, 18, 31, 32].

3. Indications for reintervention in chronic residual dissection

Deciding when to reintervene on a chronic dissection after type A repair hinges on several key indications. In the absence of formal guidelines dedicated solely to chronic dissection, most experts have historically deferred to established aortic aneurysm criteria (with some adjustments for the dissection context) [56]. The primary triggers are related to aneurysm size and growth rate, although symptoms and other complications are also critical factors. The major indications can be summarized as in **Figure 2**.

- Aneurysm diameter threshold: The most straightforward trigger for elective intervention is when the dissected aorta enlarges to a dangerous diameter. In general, an absolute diameter of 5.5 cm in the ascending or descending thoracic aorta is the classical threshold for elective repair in degenerative (nondissection) aneurysms. For chronic dissections of the descending thoracic aorta (the typical location of residual disease after type A repair), intervention is usually recommended once the aorta reaches around 5.0–5.5 cm [6–8]. Many experts favor the lower end of this range (~5.0 cm) in the setting of a chronic dissection, given that the dissection weakens the aortic wall and may pose a higher rupture risk at a smaller size. Indeed, one review noted that "reoperations for residual aortic dissections are indicated when the aortic diameter has reached the guideline threshold, i.e., 5.0 or 5.5 cm." The exact cutoff may be individualized: for example, in a patient with Marfan syndrome or a bicuspid aortic valve (genetic factors associated with connective tissue weakness), many surgeons would act at 5.0 cm or even slightly below, whereas in an older patient with no connective tissue disorder, waiting until closer to 5.5 cm might be reasonable. Ultimately, the trend is as important as the absolute number – a slightly smaller aorta that is steadily enlarging might merit repair before it ever reaches 5.5 cm.

- Rapid aortic growth: Expansion rate is a crucial indicator of impending problems. As mentioned, a growth rate greater than 10 mm/year (or >5 mm in 6 months) is generally considered a strong indication for intervention in chronic dissection. Such rapid growth suggests high wall stress or additional intimal tearing and portends rupture if left unchecked. In chronic type B dissections, aneurysmal dilation and rapid aortic growth are the most frequent indications for late treatment, and the same principle applies to residual type A dissections. Notably, growth rate can sometimes be a more sensitive marker than absolute size – for instance, an aorta expanding from 40 to 50 mm within a year is at very high risk and should be addressed rather than waiting until it definitively exceeds 5.5 cm [6, 8, 19].

- Symptoms (pain or compression): Any new symptoms attributable to the chronic dissection should prompt consideration of intervention, even if size criteria are not yet met. The classic symptom concerning for expansion is unexplained pain in the chest, back, or abdomen in a patient with known aortic dissection. Chronic

Criteria	ACC/AHA 2022	ESC 2024 (PAAD)	EACTS/STS 2024
Maximum diameter	Root/ascending 5.0–5.5 cm (lower in selected patients) Descending typically ≥6.0 cm Lower in chronic dissection by case	Generally 5.0–5.5 cm Individualized in CTD	≥55 mm (Class I, B) ≥50 mm if staged repair (Class IIa, C).
Rapid growth	≥0.5 cm/yr or ≥0.3 cm/yr over 2 yrs ≥0.3 cm/yr in HTAD/BAV	Rapid expansion indication: ~0.5 cm/yr, lower in HTAD	Risk factor for earlier repair; numeric cut-offs not fixed
Symptoms / rupture	Urgent if pain, contained leak, rupture	Urgent/emergent repair for rupture or symptoms	Emergency for rupture/contained leak (Class I).
Malperfusion	Reintervention to resolve malperfusion (endo/open)	Treat organ ischemia due to branch compromise	Treat dSINE, flow issues, address malperfusion.
HTAD / BAV	≥5.0 cm root/ascending ≥4.5 cm with high-risk HTAD	Lower thresholds based on genotype/family history.	Marfan: ≥50 mm (Class I, B) and ≥45 mm with risk (Class IIa).
Planned staged hybrid	Staging reasonable	Supports staged strategies	≥50 mm if staged plan (Class IIa, C).

Figure 2.
Comparison of aortic guidelines.

dissections are often asymptomatic until they enlarge substantially, but new-onset pain can signal rapid expansion or impending rupture and, therefore, typically warrants intervention regardless of diameter. In some cases, large chronic dissecting aneurysms can cause compressive or mass-effect symptoms – for example, hoarseness from left recurrent laryngeal nerve compression, difficulty swallowing (dysphagia) from esophageal compression, or cough and dyspnea from tracheobronchial compression. While these manifestations are less common, their presence suggests the aneurysm is anatomically significant and likely requires treatment irrespective of the absolute size.

- Malperfusion syndromes: Chronic dissections can occasionally lead to malperfusion of branch vessels, though this is more typical in the acute phase. Still, late malperfusion can occur due to gradual occlusion or compression of branch arteries by the false lumen or by thrombus. Signs such as new or refractory hypertension (from renal artery compromise), intermittent claudication, or mesenteric ischemia (e.g., postprandial abdominal pain) in a patient with chronic dissection should be taken seriously. If imaging confirms branch vessel compromise (for example, celiac artery or superior mesenteric artery narrowing by the dissection flap), intervention – either surgical or endovascular – is indicated to restore adequate perfusion. In the Marseille prospective series of residual type A dissections, about 3.5% of patients eventually underwent a distal reintervention specifically for malperfusion syndromes, even in the chronic phase. Although uncommon, this scenario is an important indication for timely reintervention to prevent end-organ damage [2, 3, 11, 37, 57].

- Aortic rupture or impending rupture: This is an emergency indication rather than an elective one. If a chronic dissection aneurysm shows imaging signs of impending rupture – such as a focal contained rupture, a crescent-shaped hyperdense area in the aortic wall on CT (the "crescent sign"), or rapid enlargement accompanied by severe pain – then immediate intervention is mandatory. Fortunately, routine surveillance is aimed at catching aneurysmal expansion before rupture occurs. Nevertheless, rupture risk rises significantly once the descending thoracic aorta diameter exceeds ~6 cm (even in chronic dissection), or at somewhat smaller sizes in patients with connective tissue disorders. Any evidence of leak or imminent rupture on imaging demands urgent surgical or endovascular repair [6–8, 18, 31, 32].

- Progressive aortic valve or root involvement: Although the focus in chronic residual dissection is usually on the distal aorta, one must not forget the proximal remnant. If the aortic root was not replaced in the initial surgery (many type A repairs involve an ascending graft with the native root left intact), that root can dilate over time, or the aortic valve may develop late insufficiency. The development of severe aortic regurgitation or a true aneurysm of the residual root (generally threshold ~5.0 cm, or lower in a Marfan patient) would be an indication for a reoperation on the proximal aorta and valve. These proximal reinterventions are less common than distal ones, but surgical series report that a smaller fraction (around 5–10%) of type A repair patients ultimately require a later root or ascending

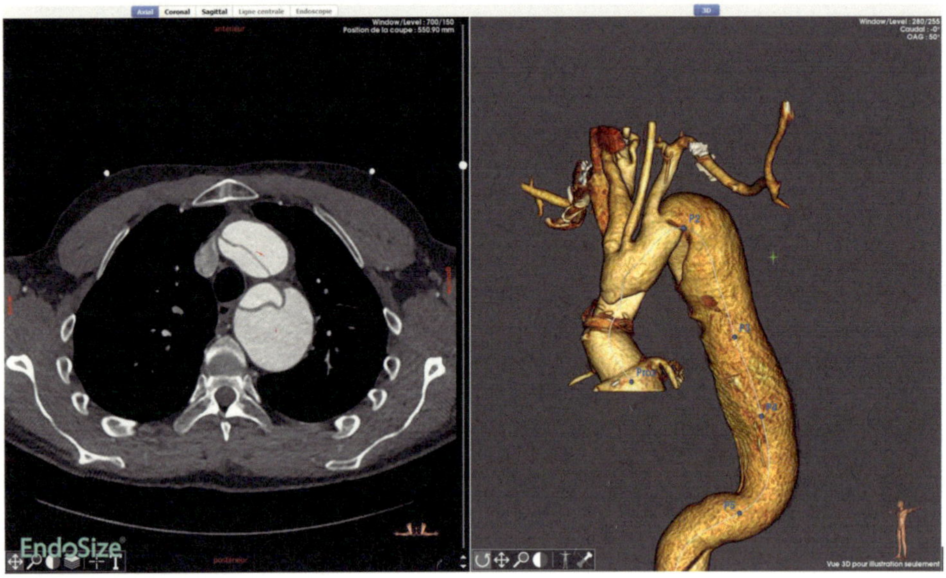

Figure 3.
Aneurysmal evolution following type A dissection treated with a hemiarch repair.

reoperation. Indications for these follow standard guidelines for aortic root aneurysm (size and growth) or symptomatic valve disease [6–8].

It is worth highlighting that the majority of reinterventions after a type A repair are on the distal aorta (arch and descending) because the initial operation addresses the ascending aorta, leaving the dissection in more distal segments (**Figure 3**). For example, one large multicenter study of 601 type A dissection patients found that 11.8% of patients underwent at least one aortic reintervention; of those, distal aortic procedures outnumbered proximal reoperations by nearly 5:1. In that study, the median time to the first reintervention was about 4.0 years after the initial repair. Other series have noted that many reinterventions occur even sooner (within 1–2 years) if aneurysmal progression is evident. In the Marseille prospective follow-up, for instance, over 80% of all distal reinterventions occurred within the first 2 years after the initial surgery. This underscores that high-risk anatomy often declares itself early, raising the question of whether some patients might benefit from a planned staged approach rather than a purely reactive strategy – an issue discussed under Timing and Strategy in **Figure 3** [6–8, 18, 31, 32].

Finally, given the complexity of these cases, decisions for reintervention should be made by a multidisciplinary aortic team (including cardiac surgeons, vascular surgeons, cardiologists, radiologists, anesthesiologists, etc.) at a center experienced in aortic pathology. Each patient's anatomy, comorbidities, and personal preferences must be weighed. For borderline cases (e.g., a~5.0cm aorta in a stable older patient), continued observation with very close follow-up may be reasonable; whereas for a younger patient or one with connective tissue disease, earlier elective intervention is favored. A team approach ensures that medical, endovascular, and surgical options are all considered, and the patient receives an individualized plan [6–8, 18, 31, 32] (**Figure 4**).

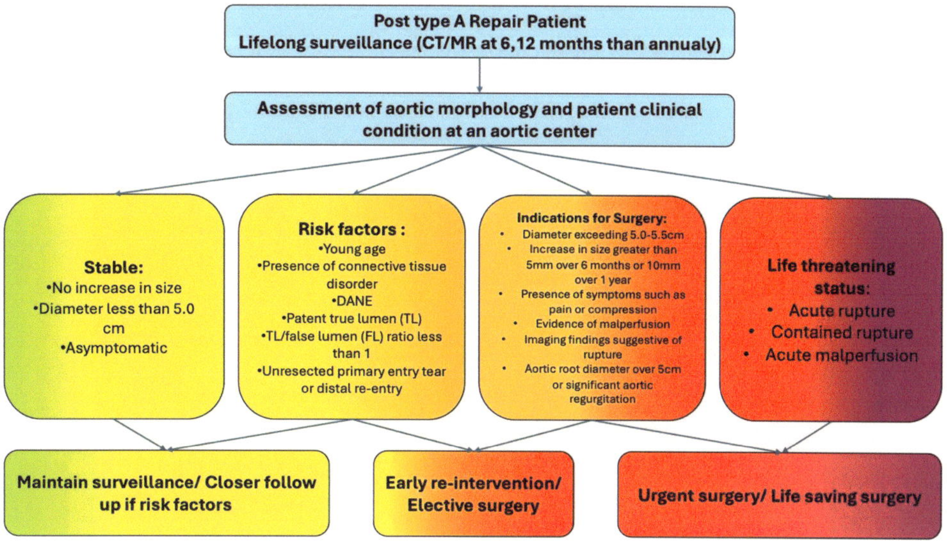

Figure 4.
Reintervention strategy algorithm.

4. Open surgical reinterventions

Open surgical repair remains the definitive treatment for many chronic dissection patients, especially those who are good surgical candidates or who have anatomy less favorable to endovascular solutions. The choice between open surgery and less invasive options depends on patient factors and the extent of disease (**Figure 5**). Situations in which a traditional open reoperation is often preferred include [4, 52, 53]

- Connective tissue disorders and young patients: In patients with Marfan syndrome, Loeys-Dietz syndrome, vascular Ehlers-Danlos syndrome, or other heritable aortopathies, open surgery is generally favored for distal aneurysm repair. These patients have fragile tissue and a propensity for continued degeneration, making durable fixation by stent grafts more challenging. A young Marfan patient with a chronically dissected descending aneurysm, for example, would likely be recommended an open repair to definitively resect the diseased segment (**Figures 6**, 7) Stent grafts in such patients have higher failure rates due to the aggressive tissue pathology [6, 8, 19].

- Very large or extensive aneurysms: If the residual dissection has led to a very large aneurysm, or if the disease spans a long segment (e.g., a thoracoabdominal aneurysm involving visceral branch vessels), an open repair may be preferred in an otherwise healthy patient. While complex endovascular solutions (such as branched or fenestrated stent grafts) exist for extensive disease, an open surgical approach can often treat all segments in one or two stages with long-term durability. In essence, beyond a certain size or extent, open surgery offers the only way to completely replace the diseased aorta and eliminate the false lumen [2, 3, 11, 37, 57, 58] (**Figure 8**).

Technique	Advantages	Limitations	Outcomes (typical elective)	Preferred Indications
Open Surgery (descending / arch / TAAA)	Definitive resection of diseased aorta Removes false lumen in treated segment Durable with low risk of late reintervention in expert centers Suitable for hostile anatomy.	Invasive (thoracotomy/sternotomy, CPB/DHCA for arch) Higher perioperative physiologic stress; risk of neurologic complications (SCI/stroke) if extensive Requires high-volume expertise	Elective mortality typically low single digits in expert centers Stroke ~2–5% (arch) Spinal cord ischemia ~3–8% for extensive descending/TAAA Excellent long-term durability.	Young patients Heritable aortopathy (Marfan/Loeys–Dietz) Very large/extensive aneurysm Failure/complications after TEVAR Anatomy unsuitable for endografts.
TEVAR (thoracic endovascular aortic repair)	Minimally invasive Shorter ICU/hospital stay Seals proximal entry tear Promotes true-lumen expansion and false-lumen thrombosis in covered segments Useful in frail/elderly.	Needs adequate landing zones Persistent distal re-entry may maintain FL Risk of endoleak/dSINE Durability depends on anatomy Device size ceiling (~40 mm) Arch geometry may be hostile.	Elective mortality ~1–5% Stroke ~0–5% (higher with arch manipulation/LSA coverage without revascularization) Spinal cord ischemia ~0–5% with long coverage Frequent need for staged distal interventions.	Older/comorbid patients Favorable proximal landing (often surgical graft) Limited thoracic disease Need for rapid stabilization Bridge in staged strategies.
Hybrid – Frozen Elephant Trunk (FET)	One-stage arch replacement with integrated descending stent Creates robust landing zone for future TEVAR Addresses arch + proximal descending simultaneously	Requires sternotomy and cerebral protection Neurologic risk (stroke/SCI) in extensive disease Often still requires second-stage distal work.	Contemporary series: low elective mortality in expert centers Stroke reported ~5–15% depending on extent Temporary SCI ~0–8% Good proximal remodeling Staged distal reintervention common	Arch + proximal descending involvement To facilitate downstream endovascular completion Complex arch tears/DANE Patients suitable for open arch
Hybrid – Arch Debranching + TEVAR	Avoids redo full arch under circulatory arrest Expands proximal landing zone to Zone 0–2 Useful in high-risk resternotomy Customizable to anatomy	Two components (surgical bypasses + endograft) Risk of graft infection/occlusion Carries stroke risk from arch manipulation Careful planning for LSA/carotid revascularization.	Elective mortality generally low in experienced teams Stroke ~3–8% reported SCI risk depends on length of thoracic coverage Good durability but surveillance for endoleak required.	Unfavorable arch anatomy for simple TEVAR High risk for full arch replacement Needing to land proximally without circulatory arrest Staged strategies

Figure 5.
Evaluation of different treatment methods.

DOI: http://dx.doi.org/10.5772/intechopen.1013577

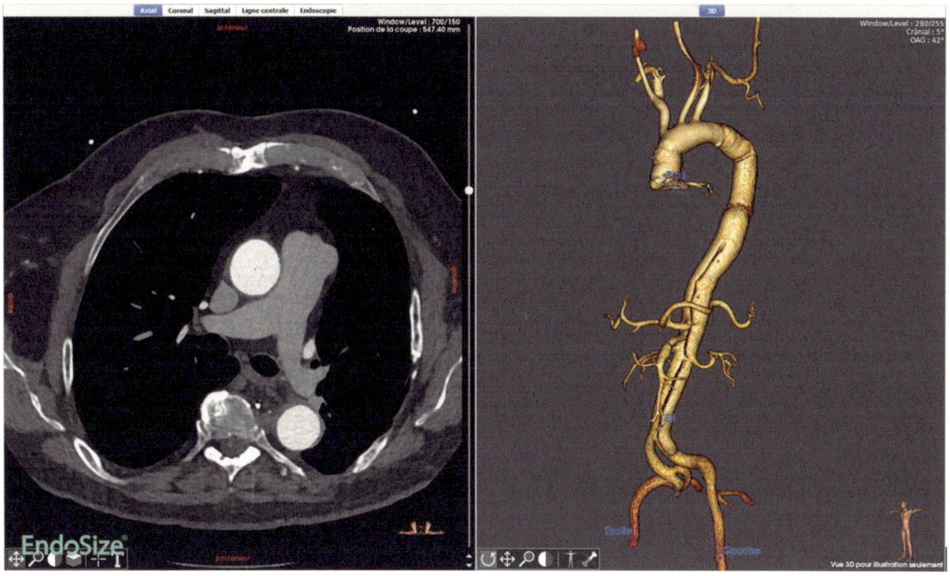

Figure 6.
CT scan and 3D reconstruction after open descending aortic repair.

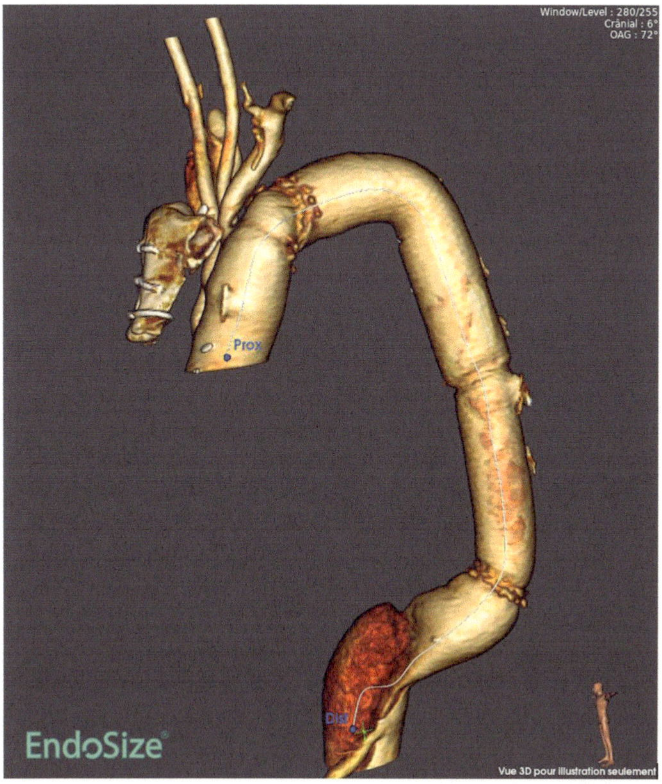

Figure 7.
3D reconstruction after total open descending aortic repair. Patient with a history of arch replacement using a conventional elephant trunk technique for a type A dissection surgery.

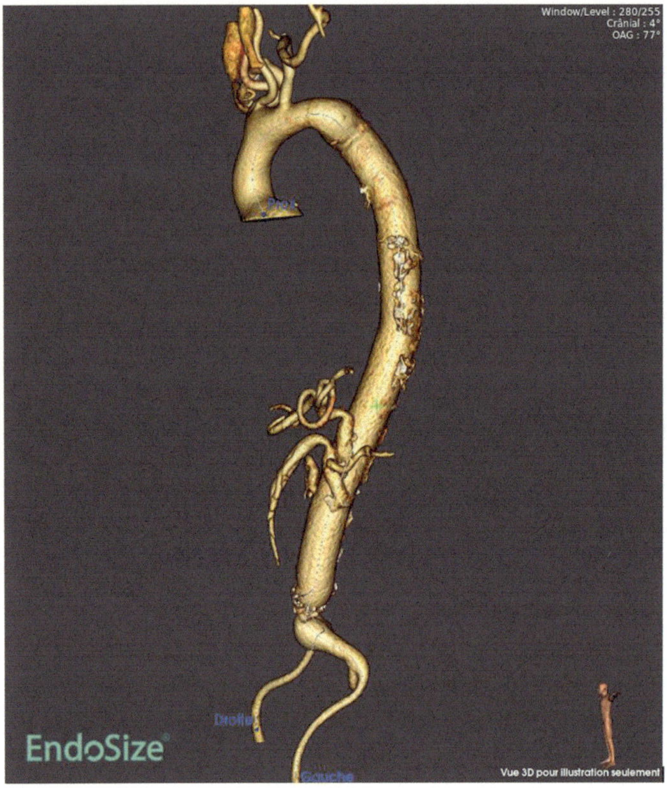

Figure 8.
3D reconstruction showing results after open repair of a thoraco-abdominal aneurysm.

- Prior failed endovascular repair: If the patient has already undergone a distal aortic stent-graft (thoracic endovascular aortic repair [TEVAR]) as a previous intervention and now presents with complications (such as a persistent endoleak, continued false lumen perfusion, or new aneurysm formation distal to the stent), an open conversion may be required. In some cases, the endograft can be left in place and the aorta replaced around it; in others, the graft may need to be partially or fully removed. Prior endovascular treatment failure is a strong indication to opt for open surgery to definitively address the problem [2, 3, 11, 37, 57].

Outcomes of open reinterventions: Historically, reoperations on the aorta carried substantial risks, but outcomes have improved significantly in experienced high-volume centers. Elective open descending and thoracoabdominal repairs for chronic dissection can now often be performed with <10% operative mortality in many expert centers. For example, the Kawasaki Aortic Center in Japan (known for a "no turn-down" policy for even complex cases) reported excellent results in 492 patients who underwent open descending thoracic aortic replacement for chronic dissection: An early mortality of only 2.0%, a stroke rate of 3.5%, and a spinal cord injury rate of 6.1%. Among a low-risk subset of those patients (age <70, elective cases), outcomes were even better – operative mortality ~0.4% and stroke ~1.5%. Five-year survival after open repair in that series was about 87%, and only ~8% of patients required any further aortic intervention by 5 years. These results suggest that open surgical repair of the chronic dissected aorta can be a gold-standard, durable solution in appropriate patients. Similarly, an Italian multicenter study focusing on the frozen elephant trunk (FET) technique in chronic residual dissections reported 0% 30-day mortality in 28 patients, with 2-year survival ~92%. However, they did note significant morbidity: About 14% had a stroke, and 7% had a temporary spinal cord deficit, reflecting the extensive nature of the procedure. Notably, in that series, the freedom from downstream reintervention at 2 years was only ~59% – meaning a substantial portion of patients required additional procedures later (often planned second-stage interventions) despite the FET, underscoring that a staged approach is frequently necessary [23, 41, 45, 58–63, 65].

Open arch and descending reoperations have unique hazards, particularly neurological complications. Redo sternotomy and arch replacement carry a risk of stroke due to arch vessel manipulation or aortic debris, and spinal cord ischemia can occur if the repair extends into the descending thoracic aorta (especially if intercostal arteries are sacrificed). Techniques to mitigate these risks include meticulous cerebral protection strategies during arch reoperations (such as the use of deep hypothermic circulatory arrest or selective antegrade cerebral perfusion to protect the brain while the arch is repaired) and spinal cord protection measures during extensive descending/thoracoabdominal repairs (cerebrospinal fluid drainage to improve spinal perfusion, moderate hypothermia, reimplantation of critical intercostal arteries when feasible, perioperative hemoglobin thresholds, etc.). Modern refinements like the “branch-first” or “distal-first” approaches have been described to reduce organ ischemia times. For instance, Estrera et al. have popularized a “distal-first” technique in chronic descending/thoracoabdominal repairs, where the distal anastomosis is constructed first under left heart bypass (thereby perfusing the distal aorta throughout), and then the proximal anastomosis is done – ensuring continuous perfusion to critical branches for a longer duration. Such strategies have helped drive down the morbidity of open surgery. Still, even in the best hands, patients must be counseled about a roughly 5–10% risk of major complications (stroke, renal failure, or paralysis) in elective open reoperations. For urgent or emergency reinterventions (e.g., for impending rupture), the risk profile is higher due to suboptimal conditions [28, 46].

In summary, open surgery offers the advantage of complete excision of the diseased aorta and obliteration of the false lumen, which generally eliminates the problem of recurrent aneurysm in that segment. Long-term surveillance is still required (since other untreated segments of the aorta can dilate later), but a successful open repair tends to have a low recurrence of false lumen flow in the repaired segment. Thus, for low-risk patients with suitable anatomy, many centers still consider open reintervention as a first-line choice – especially if the anatomy is too complex for a reliable endovascular fix. On the other hand, for patients with significant comorbidities or anatomy that is favorable for stenting, less invasive options are very attractive, as discussed next [6–8, 18, 31, 32].

5. Endovascular and hybrid interventions

The advent of TEVAR has revolutionized the treatment of distal aortic pathology over the last two decades. In the context of chronic aortic dissection, TEVAR offers a minimally invasive option that avoids the morbidity of a major open thoracotomy or redo sternotomy. The principle of TEVAR in dissection is to deploy covered stent-grafts inside the true lumen to seal the proximal tear, induce false lumen thrombosis, and stabilize (or shrink) the aneurysmal aorta (**Figure 9**). TEVAR has become an established therapy for chronic type B (distal) dissections and is increasingly applied to residual dissections after type A as well, when anatomy and patient factors are suitable. In fact, the INSTEAD-XL trial demonstrated that in uncomplicated chronic type B dissection, elective TEVAR (plus medical therapy) led to better aortic remodeling and fewer aorta-related deaths at five years compared to medical therapy alone. While no such randomized trial exists specifically for residual type A dissections, by analogy, many experts believe that preemptively stabilizing the chronically dissected distal aorta with TEVAR can prevent late complications and improve long-term outcomes in these patients [1–5, 64–66].

Anatomic requirements and considerations: Successful TEVAR depends on having adequate "landing zones" – segments of relatively normal (nondissected), stable aorta where the stent-graft can securely seal. In chronic posttype A dissection cases, the proximal landing zone is often the surgical graft in the ascending/arch. If the surgical repair included a hemiarch replacement (distal anastomosis in the midarch), the graft extends to the proximal arch, and a stent can be landed just distal to the left common carotid artery (Zone 2) or across the left subclavian artery (Zone 3), if needed. If only

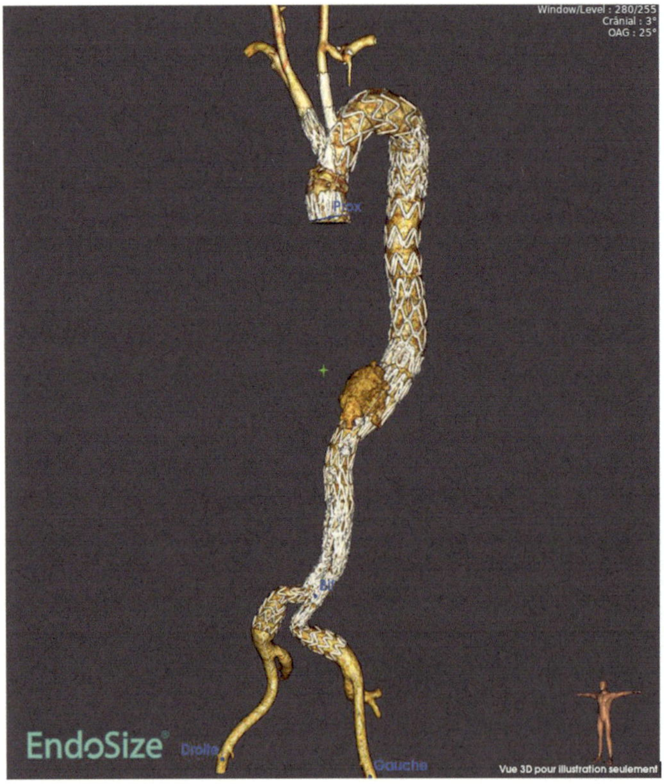

Figure 9.
3D reconstruction following a total endovascular repair.

the ascending aorta was replaced and the intimal tear is at the original distal anastomosis near the brachiocephalic artery, then achieving a good proximal seal may require covering the arch vessels (Zone 0/1) or using branched endograft technology, which is more complex (see Hybrid approaches below). Key criteria for TEVAR include [6–8]:

Landing zone length: Ideally, at least ~2 cm of relatively straight, nondissected aorta is needed proximally (and distally) for the stent graft to seal without endoleak. Often, achieving a good proximal landing zone necessitates covering the left subclavian artery; in elective cases, a left carotid-subclavian bypass can be performed prior to TEVAR to preserve perfusion to the left arm if the subclavian artery will be covered [6–8].

Aortic diameter: The proximal landing zone (often the surgical graft or native arch segment) must be within the size range of available stent grafts. Most thoracic stent grafts can accommodate diameters up to about 40 mm. Surgical grafts are usually <30 mm, which is ideal; but if the residual arch is aneurysmal (e.g. >40 mm; a TEVAR alone will not suffice without treating the arch (open or with a branched device). Oversizing of the stent (typically 10–20% diameter oversize) is required in dissection to ensure a seal in the true lumen, but excessive oversizing can risk inducing a new intimal tear or retrograde dissection [6–8].

Arch geometry: Sharp angulation or a "gothic arch" configuration can pose challenges for endograft navigation and sealing. Severe arch tortuosity or circumferential atherosclerotic plaque increases the risk of endograft malapposition or provoking a retrograde dissection from the graft's proximal edge. In such cases, an open arch or hybrid approach might be safer.

Access vessels: The femoral and iliac arteries must be large and healthy enough to accommodate the delivery sheath of the thoracic stent graft (which can be 20–25 French, roughly 6–8 mm in diameter). In patients with small or diseased iliac arteries, surgical exposure or enlargement (or the use of a surgical conduit graft sewn to the iliac artery) may be necessary to introduce the device.

When these anatomical criteria are met, TEVAR can be very effective in the chronic dissection setting. The procedure usually involves inserting the stent-graft via the femoral artery (sometimes the iliac or axillary artery) and positioning it to cover the primary intimal tear (often at or just distal to the left subclavian artery origin in residual type A cases). By sealing off the proximal entry tear, blood flow into the false lumen is reduced, ideally leading to thrombosis of the false lumen in the stent-covered segments. This relieves pressure on the aortic wall and often halts or reverses aneurysm growth. Over time, the treated segment of the aorta may even shrink as remodeling occurs [1–5].

Outcomes of TEVAR in chronic dissection: Numerous series have shown that TEVAR in chronic dissections can be performed with high technical success and relatively low immediate morbidity. The risk of paraplegia (spinal cord ischemia) in chronic dissection TEVAR is lower than in extensive open surgery, but it is not negligible if long segments of the aorta (especially covering multiple intercostal artery zones) are stented. Stroke risk is also present (typically 0–5%), depending on arch manipulation and coverage of arch branches. In properly selected patients, however, the 30-day mortality of elective TEVAR for chronic dissection aneurysms is often reported in the low single digits (around 1–5%). For example, a meta-analysis of TEVAR for chronic type B dissection found early mortality ~1.6% (though this included various series). TEVAR's less invasive nature often translates to shorter hospital stays and faster recovery compared to open surgery [6–8].

One challenge in chronic dissection TEVAR is that closing the primary tear may not thrombose the entire false lumen if there are multiple distal reentry tears or if the false lumen is already large and pressurized. In such cases, TEVAR can halt expansion in the thoracic segment, but the abdominal aorta may continue to enlarge (so-called distal stent graft-induced new entry, or dSINE, can also occur at the end of the stent). To address this, sometimes a staged approach with distal extension of the stent-graft or additional interventions (e.g., coil embolization of the false lumen or a distal surgical replacement) may be needed down the line [1–5].

Hybrid approaches: For some patients, neither an isolated open surgery nor a simple TEVAR is ideal. Hybrid strategies combine open and endovascular techniques, either concurrently or in stages, to tailor the treatment. One common hybrid scenario in chronic type A residual dissection is the arch debranching plus TEVAR approach: An open surgical bypass is created to reroute blood flow to one or more supra-aortic vessels (for example, a bypass from the ascending aorta to the left carotid and subclavian arteries), and then an endograft is placed into the arch/descending aorta, covering the origins of those vessels. This effectively achieves an arch repair without a full arch replacement, avoiding the need for deep hypothermic arrest. Hybrid arch repair is an option for patients who cannot undergo a conventional open arch replacement but who have suitable anatomy for endografting once the head vessels are rerouted. Another scenario is the staged elephant trunk: For example, performing an open arch replacement with a FET (a stent-graft prosthesis frozen into the descending aorta), then later landing additional endografts or performing abdominal aortic surgery as needed [6–10].

In recent years, dedicated hybrid graft devices (which include a sewn arch graft with an integrated stent for the proximal descending aorta) have been employed in chronic residual dissection cases, with promising results (**Figure 10**). Branched endografts for the arch (with branches for great vessels) are also under development and in early use, potentially allowing totally endovascular arch repairs in the future. At present, these remain specialized techniques reserved for high-risk or anatomically complex cases [6–8].

In summary, endovascular repair has become a game-changing option, enabling treatment of descending (and even arch) aneurysms with dramatically lower immediate morbidity than open surgery. Hybrid approaches capitalize on the strengths of both modalities, tailoring the treatment to the patient's anatomy and condition (for example, arch debranching plus TEVAR to avoid a risky redo sternotomy). No single approach is universally best – often the multidisciplinary team will deploy multiple different tools over the course of a patient's lifetime as the disease evolves [6–8].

6. Timing and strategy: How to approach reinterventions

A crucial aspect of managing chronic dissections after type A repair is the timing – not only when to intervene based on the aortic pathology's progression, but also how to time and stage interventions if a multistep approach is anticipated. Several scenarios and strategic considerations can be outlined (**Figure 11**).

Immediate or early postrepair intervention: In certain cases, the distal aorta is already significantly diseased at the time of the initial acute type A surgery. For instance, if the descending thoracic aorta is acutely dissected and measures, for example, 4.5–5.0 cm with a large false lumen during the acute episode, some

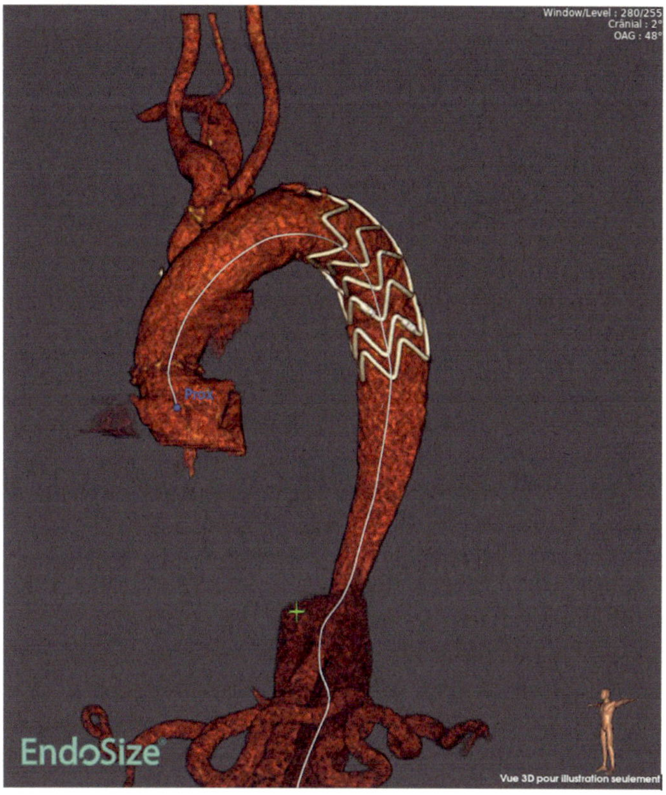

Figure 10.
3D reconstruction following aortic repair using an FET prosthesis.

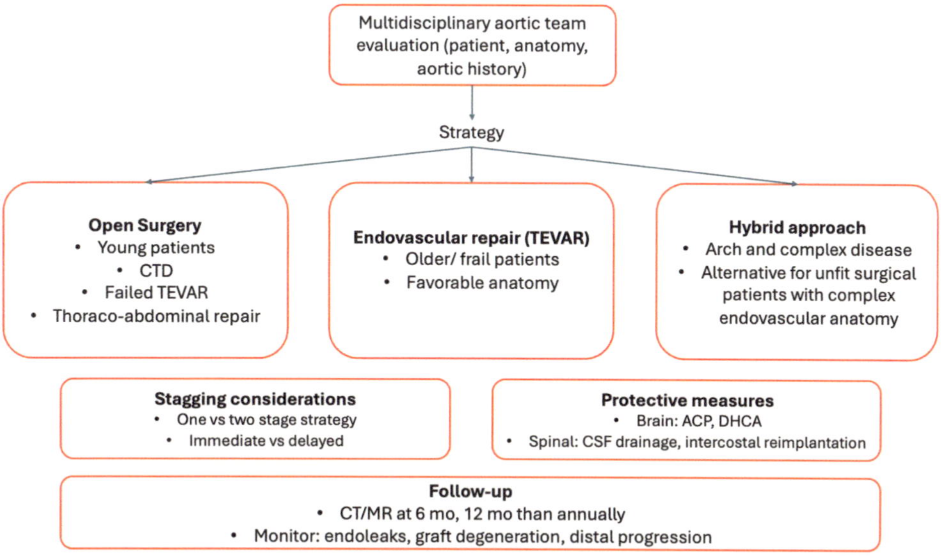

Figure 11.
Aortic intervention planning considerations.

surgeons opt to perform a more extensive initial repair (such as a total arch replacement with a FET) to proactively address the distal aorta in one setting. Others may prefer to first stabilize the patient by completing the ascending repair and then perform a planned second-stage procedure shortly after (within days to a few weeks), once the patient has recovered from the initial operation but before the dissection fully enters a chronic phase. This second stage could be a TEVAR or an open descending repair, done in the subacute period (e.g., two to eight weeks postop) to induce false lumen thrombosis and favorable remodeling before significant scarring or aneurysm expansion occurs. Early TEVAR after type A repair (sometimes called a "provisional extension to induce complete attachment" or PETTICOAT approach, when a bare stent in the abdominal aorta is also used) has been attempted in some high-risk cases. Some experts recommend waiting at least a few days to a couple of weeks after the acute surgery to reduce operative risk (allowing inflammation to subside). It's important to note that routine immediate second-stage stenting for everyone is not standard practice; it's reserved for those with concerning distal anatomy at baseline. Most patients, if their distal aorta is not severely enlarged, will enter a period of surveillance after the acute repair, unless clear indications for early intervention emerge [9–16].

Elective versus urgent versus emergency timing: Once a chronic dissection aneurysm meets the criteria for intervention (size or symptoms), the goal is to perform the reintervention electively, if at all possible, because outcomes are best when done in a controlled, nonemergent setting. For example, an asymptomatic 5.5 cm chronic dissecting aneurysm should be scheduled for repair in a timely fashion (on the order of weeks to a couple of months, not waiting indefinitely). If there are concerning symptoms, such as pain, the timeline accelerates – many would consider that a semi-urgent indication (intervene within days to one to two weeks), since pain can herald instability. A frank contained rupture or critical malperfusion constitutes an emergency, requiring immediate intervention (within hours), much like an acute dissection. Thus, "when to reintervene" can range from right now (in a rupture scenario) to potentially never (if a patient's residual dissection remains stable under threshold and they eventually die of unrelated causes). In practice, the majority of elective reinterventions tend to occur in the 1–10 year window after the initial surgery. Notably, analyses show the incidence of reintervention plateaus after ~10 years postrepair – those whose aortas have remained stable for a decade may be less likely to require later intervention (though not guaranteed) [11, 13].

One-stage versus two-stage repairs: For extensive disease involving multiple aortic segments (e.g., a residual dissection aneurysm extending from the arch all the way to the abdominal aorta), a single intervention may not be sufficient or safe to address the entire pathology at once. Traditionally, such extensive repairs were done in two open stages (e.g., an arch replacement first, then a separate open descending/thoracoabdominal surgery later). With modern techniques like the FET, many arch and proximal descending issues can be handled in one stage, with any remaining distal work tackled in a planned second stage (either via TEVAR or an open abdominal/thoracoabdominal repair). In chronic dissection scenarios, a staged hybrid approach is common: For instance, perform an arch replacement with FET now, then follow up with a second-stage TEVAR or open abdominal aortic repair months or years later. The optimal interval between stages depends on the urgency – it could be within the same hospitalization (if anatomy demands rapid completion to prevent rupture), or it could be spaced out over months to years if the remaining segment can be safely observed until it reaches an intervention threshold. Aneurysm growth rates can inform timing: If after stage 1 the downstream aorta is, say, 45 mm and stable, one might simply monitor until it grows to ~55 mm over a couple of years before doing stage 2. On the other hand, if at the time of stage 1 the distal aorta is already large (e.g., 60 mm), a second stage should be done relatively soon (some centers even plan it in the same hospital stay after the patient recovers from stage 1, particularly if there are concerns about losing the patient to follow-up) [11–16].

Impact of initial repair extent: It's worth noting that the extent of the initial type A repair can influence the timing and likelihood of later interventions. Patients who only had the ascending aorta replaced (a supracoronary graft) and were left with a dissected arch have a higher chance of needing an arch or descending intervention within a few years. In contrast, those who had a more aggressive acute repair (such as a total arch replacement with FET) might go longer without reintervention. An analysis in JACC noted that roughly 10–20% of patients require reintervention in the first 10 years, and these often correlate with less extensive initial repairs and residual distal false lumen flow. Current guidelines encourage performing at least an open distal anastomosis into the arch (hemiarch repair) during acute type A surgery to eliminate the intimal tear in the arch, rather than doing a short ascending graft that leaves a tear at the arch – this strategy reduces the early distal reentry tear issue. Nevertheless, even a hemiarch leaves the descending dissection in place, so late interventions may still occur. Some experts advocate for a routine total arch + FET in acute type A cases for select patients to minimize later problems, but this comes at the price of a higher initial operative risk. Observational data suggest that doing a more extensive arch upfront can reduce but not eliminate reinterventions; and importantly, the immediate survival is generally better with a more limited repair in an emergency setting. Thus, many centers still stand on the side of a conservative proximal repair during the acute dissection, accepting the possibility of a second-stage elective distal repair in the future, rather than jeopardizing the initial survival [11–13].

In practice, once a chronic dissection patient is approaching intervention criteria, careful planning is undertaken. Detailed imaging – often including 3D reconstructions and centerline measurements on CTA – is performed to strategize the exact approach. If an endovascular repair is planned, imaging of the entire vascular tree (aorta and access vessels, plus cerebral circulation if arch work is involved) is needed to ensure feasibility. If open surgery is planned, one must assess factors like the location of prior grafts (to plan aortic clamp sites or anastomoses), the condition of critical branch vessels (coronary bypass grafts, carotid arteries, etc.), and any anatomical changes since the initial surgery (e.g., patent coronary bypass grafts from a prior CABG could influence the approach). It is often beneficial to have backup plans: For example, if a TEVAR is intended but intraoperatively the landing zone is found to be inadequate, the team should be prepared to convert to an open solution or use adjunct techniques (like a chimney graft or scallop) to salvage the repair. These complex reinterventions are best approached with flexibility and a full armamentarium of skills available [11–16].

7. Outcomes and considerations after reintervention

The ultimate goals of reintervening on chronic dissections are to prolong life and relieve symptoms by preventing aortic rupture or other catastrophic events. The encouraging news is that, in experienced centers, patients who undergo these secondary interventions tend to have good long-term outcomes, especially when done electively. A contemporary study from the University of Pittsburgh found that patients requiring reintervention after a type A dissection repair had similar long-term survival to those who did not need a reintervention, after adjusting for baseline differences. In that study, the 10-year survival did not significantly differ between the reintervention group and the no-reintervention group, implying that timely aortic reoperations (when indicated) can be performed without compromising life expectancy. The operative mortality for the reinterventions in that series was around 5–6%, and importantly, these interventions prevented what likely would have been fatal outcomes (aneurysm ruptures or dissection extensions) if left untreated. In other words, the reinterventions achieved their purpose of averting aortic catastrophes, justifying the risk [11–16].

Long-term surveillance must, of course, continue even after a reintervention. If an open repair is done, any remaining distal aorta (or other unresected segments) still requires periodic monitoring. If an endograft is placed, annual imaging is mandatory to check for endoleaks, stent migration, or new aneurysm formation beyond the stent. In many cases of residual dissection, an intervention may solve one part of the aorta but leave another segment under observation (e.g., treat the thoracic aorta, continue to watch the abdominal aorta). Thus, the patient essentially reenters a life-long surveillance program similar to after the initial repair – though hopefully with a more stable aorta postintervention [11–16].

One interesting finding from larger series is that a successful reintervention can significantly promote false lumen thrombosis and positive aortic remodeling. In the Marseille 5-year follow-up study, for example, after distal interventions (hybrid arch or branched endografts), over 85% of patients achieved complete false lumen thrombosis in the treated thoracic segment. This positive remodeling is crucial because it means the risk of further expansion in that segment is greatly reduced. However, one must remember that partial thrombosis of the false lumen beyond the treated segment can still occur and needs observation – in chronic dissection, a partially thrombosed false lumen in untreated segments has been associated with continued expansion of those segments [11–16].

Another consideration is the quality of life after these interventions. Generally, patients who undergo a successful elective repair of a chronic dissection aneurysm are relieved of the constant anxiety about an impending rupture, and they often return to a good functional status. Those treated with endovascular stents recover particularly quickly – many are discharged home in just a few days and back to normal activities within a couple of weeks. Patients undergoing open reoperations have a longer recovery (similar to the recovery after their initial type A surgery); but if the procedure is elective and uncomplicated, even these patients can often return to an active life within a couple of months. Most importantly, all patients require continued risk factor management: Strict blood pressure control remains essential even after the aorta is repaired, both to protect the new grafts or stents and to safeguard any remaining natural aorta from further degeneration [6–8].

It should also be noted that some patients will undergo multiple reinterventions over their lifetime. For instance, a patient with a connective tissue disorder might have an acute type A repair in their 30s, then perhaps an arch or descending procedure in their 40s, then maybe a thoracoabdominal or abdominal aortic repair in their 50s, and so on. Each segmental replacement extends their survival and can be done safely in modern times. There are reports of patients having 3–4 major aortic surgeries at different times – essentially a serial replacement of the entire aorta over years – with good outcomes. This underscores that, with current techniques, even very complex aortic disease can be managed in stages; the key is to intervene before acute disasters happen, performing elective fixes of each segment as it becomes indicated [17–21].

8. Conclusion

Chronic aortic dissections following a type A repair represent a significant management challenge, but one that can be successfully navigated with vigilant surveillance and timely intervention. Approximately half of the patients who survive an acute type A dissection will develop aneurysmal degeneration in the residual dissected aorta over the subsequent years, and a substantial subset will require a secondary procedure to prevent rupture or other late complications. The decision of when to reintervene hinges on reaching critical size (generally ~5.0–5.5 cm in the chronic phase), rapid expansion, or the development of symptoms, and should always be individualized based on patient factors and detailed imaging findings. Early recognition of high-risk features (patent false lumen, large initial aortic diameter, connective tissue disease, etc.) allows clinicians to anticipate problems and plan reinterventions proactively – sometimes even before traditional thresholds are crossed [11–16].

In terms of how to reintervene, modern aortic care offers a spectrum of options, from conventional open surgery to cutting-edge endovascular therapies, often used in a complementary fashion. Open surgical reoperations – including arch and descending replacements – continue to be the definitive solution for many patients (especially the young and low-risk) with excellent outcomes in expert hands. Meanwhile, endovascular repair (TEVAR) has emerged as a transformative option for others, enabling treatment of descending (and even arch) aneurysms with dramatically lower immediate morbidity. Hybrid approaches combine the strengths of both, tailoring the treatment to the patient's unique anatomy and condition (for example, arch debranching plus TEVAR to avoid a high-risk resternotomy). There is no one-size-fits-all solution – the multidisciplinary aortic team must weigh the trade-offs of each approach, and in many cases, multiple different interventions will be employed over the patient's lifetime [6–8].

Crucially, the management of chronic postdissection patients does not end with the intervention. Lifelong follow-up remains essential, both to monitor any remaining dissected aorta and to ensure that any repairs (grafts or stents) continue to function properly. The encouraging reality is that, with vigilant surveillance and appropriately timed reinterventions, patients can enjoy excellent long-term survival and quality of life. In specialized centers, late mortality from aortic causes has become relatively low, as nearly every potential complication can be anticipated and addressed either prophylactically or at an early stage. Advances on the horizon – such as off-the-shelf branched stent-grafts for the arch and ascending aorta, improved imaging biomarkers for detecting high-risk dissection features, and perhaps medical therapies that slow aneurysm progression – hold promise for even better outcomes in the future [11–16].

In conclusion, the management of chronic aortic dissections after type A repair is a prime example of individualized cardiovascular care. It requires a marriage of meticulous medical management, high-end imaging surveillance, sound judgment on timing, and mastery of complex surgical and endovascular techniques. When done well, reinterventions are not a "failure" of the initial repair but rather an integral part of the patient's therapeutic journey – one that ultimately extends life and prevents the horrific complications that untreated chronic dissections can cause. By remaining proactive and patient-centric in our approach, we can ensure that patients who survive an acute type A dissection not only are saved in the short run but also are protected in the long run from the shadow that the dissection casts on their aorta. As emerging data show, a strategy of timely reintervention can yield excellent survival and a low rate of aorta-related deaths, offering hope that these patients can live out a near-normal lifespan free from further aortic catastrophe [5, 7, 8, 11–16, 22–26].

Acknowledgments

The authors acknowledge the assistance of artificial intelligence–based tools (ChatGPT, OpenAI) in supporting the drafting and language refinement of this manuscript. The content, structure, and scientific interpretation remain the sole responsibility of the authors, who carefully reviewed and validated all sections.

Author details

Jacques Tomasi*, Pierre Escrig and Jean-Philippe Verhoye
Department of Thoracic and Cardio-Vascular Surgery, Aortic Surgery Unit (Rennes Aortic Center), University Hospital of Rennes, Rennes, France

*Address all correspondence to: jacques.tomasi@chu-rennes.fr

References

[1] An KR, de Mestral C, Tam DY, Qiu F, Ouzounian M, Lindsay TF, et al. Surveillance imaging following acute type A aortic dissection. Journal of the American College of Cardiology 2021;**78**:1863–1871

[2] Puthumana J, Vassallo P, Hoel A, Malaisrie SC, Mehta C. Surveillance following acute type A aortic dissection: The need for long-term clinical oversight. Journal of the American College of Cardiology. 2022;**79**(10):e205

[3] Fleischmann D, Afifi RO, Casanegra AI, Elefteriades JA, Gleason TG, Hanneman K, et al. Imaging and surveillance of chronic aortic dissection: A scientific statement from the American Heart Association. Circulation: Cardiovascular Imaging. 2022;**15**(3):e000075

[4] Heuts S, Schalla S, Ramaekers MJFG, Bidar E, Mihl C, Wildberger JE, et al. Imaging surveillance for complications after primary surgery for type A aortic dissection. Heart 2022;**109**:96–101

[5] Lescan M. Anatomical feasibility of the total endovascular aortic arch repair —and what lies beyond. European Journal of Cardio-Thoracic Surgery. 2022;**62**(3):ezac296

[6] Isselbacher EM, Preventza O, Hamilton Black J, Augoustides JG, Beck AW, Bolen MA, et al. 2022 ACC/AHA guideline for the diagnosis and management of aortic disease: A report of the American Heart Association/American College of Cardiology Joint Committee on clinical practice guidelines. Circulation 2022;**146**:e334–482

[7] Mazzolai L, Teixido-Tura G, Lanzi S, Boc V, Bossone E, Brodmann M, et al. 2024 ESC guidelines for the management of peripheral arterial and aortic diseases. European Heart Journal 2024;**45**:3538–3700

[8] Czerny M, Grabenwöger M, Berger T, Aboyans V, Della Corte A, et al. EACTS/STS guidelines for diagnosing and treating acute and chronic syndromes of the aortic organ. The Annals of Thoracic Surgery 2024;**118**:5–115

[9] Lombardi JV, Hughes GC, Appoo JJ, Bavaria JE, Beck AW, Cambria RP, et al. Society for Vascular Surgery (SVS) and Society of Thoracic Surgeons (STS) reporting standards for type B aortic dissections. Journal of Vascular Surgery 2020;**71**:I350–6

[10] Geirsson A, Bavaria JE, Swarr D, Keane MG, Woo YJ, Szeto WY, et al. Fate of the residual distal and proximal aorta after acute type a dissection repair using a contemporary surgical reconstruction algorithm. The Annals of Thoracic Surgery. 2007;**84**(6): 1955–1964. discussion 1955-1964

[11] Halstead JC, Meier M, Etz C, Spielvogel D, Bodian C, Wurm M, et al. The fate of the distal aorta after repair of acute type A aortic dissection. The Journal of Thoracic and Cardiovascular Surgery 2007;**133**:127–135

[12] Kirsch M, Soustelle C, Houël R, Hillion ML, Loisance D. Risk factor analysis for proximal and distal reoperations after surgery for acute type A aortic dissection. The Journal of Thoracic and Cardiovascular Surgery. 2002;**123**(2):318–325

[13] Concistrè G, Casali G, Santaniello E, Montalto A, Fiorani B, Dell'Aquila A, et al. Reoperation after surgical correction of acute type A aortic dissection: Risk factor analysis. The Annals of Thoracic Surgery 2012;**93**:450–455

[14] Fattouch K, Sampognaro R, Navarra E, Caruso M, Pisano C, Coppola G, et al. Long-term results after repair of type a acute aortic dissection according to false lumen patency. The Annals of Thoracic Surgery 2009;**88**:1244–1250

[15] Tsai TT, Evangelista A, Nienaber CA, Myrmel T, Meinhardt G, Cooper JV, et al. Partial thrombosis of the false lumen in patients with acute type B aortic dissection. New England Journal of Medicine 2007;**357**:349–359

[16] Igarashi T, Sato Y, Satokawa H, Takase S, Iwai-Takano M, Seto Y, et al. Ratio of the false lumen to the true lumen is associated with long-term prognosis after surgical repair of acute type A aortic dissection. JTCVS Open. 2022;**10**:75–84

[17] Yamane Y, Oshima S, Ishiko K, Okiyama M, Hirokami T, Hirai Y, et al. Descending thoracic aortic repair outcomes for chronic aortic dissection: A single-centre experience. Interactive CardioVascular and Thoracic Surgery. 2022;**35**(4):ivac233

[18] Malvindi PG, van Putte BP, Sonker U, Heijmen RH, Schepens MAAM, Morshuis WJ. Reoperation after acute type a aortic dissection repair: A series of 104 patients. The Annals of Thoracic Surgery. 2013;**95**(3):922–927

[19] Ohira S, Malekan R, Kai M, Goldberg JB, Laskowski I, De La Pena C, et al. Aortic reoperation after prior acute type A aortic dissection repair: Don't despair the repair. The Annals of Thoracic Surgery 2023;**116**:43–50

[20] Park K-H, Lim C, Choi JH, Chung E, Choi SI, Chun EJ, et al. Midterm change of descending aortic false lumen after repair of acute type I dissection. The Annals of Thoracic Surgery 2009;**87**:103–108

[21] Kölbel T, Lohrenz C, Kieback A, Diener H, Debus ES, Larena-Avellaneda A. Distal false lumen occlusion in aortic dissection with a homemade extra-large vascular plug: The candy-plug technique. Journal of Endovascular Therapy. 2013;**20**(4):484–489

[22] Leshnower BG. Better candy for the false lumen. The Journal of Thoracic and Cardiovascular Surgery. 2018;**155**(5):1973

[23] Tsagakis K, Pacini D, Grabenwöger M, Borger MA, Goebel N, Hemmer W, et al. Results of frozen elephant trunk from the international E-vita open registry. Annals of Cardiothoracic Surgery 2020;**9**:178–188

[24] Tsagakis K, Kempfert J, Zierer A, Martens A, Dohle DS, Castiglioni A, et al. E-vita OPEN NEO in the treatment of acute or chronic aortic pathologies: First interim results of the NEOS study. European Journal of Cardio-Thoracic Surgery. 2024;**65**(6)

[25] Porto A, Omnes V, Bartoli MA, Azogui R, Resseguier N, De Masi M, et al. Reintervention of residual aortic dissection after type A aortic repair: Results of a prospective follow-up at 5 years. Journal of Clinical Medicine 2023;**12**:2363

[26] Kimura N, Itoh S, Yuri K, Adachi K, Matsumoto H, Yamaguchi A,

et al. Reoperation for enlargement of the distal aorta after initial surgery for acute type A aortic dissection. The Journal of Thoracic and Cardiovascular Surgery. 2015;**149**(2):S91–S98.e1

[27] El-Andari R, Fialka NM, Alshehri A, Hassanabad AF, Bozso SJ, Moon MC. Distal anastomotic new entry tears and aortic remodeling following type A dissection repair: A systematic review. JTCVS Open. 2025;**23**:89–100

[28] Ahmad R-A, Marway P, Campello Jorge CA, Monaghan K, Satija D, Ling C, et al. Distal anastomosis new entry tear in acute type A aortic dissection: A risk factor for distal aortic reoperation. JTCVS Open. 2025;**24**:77–84

[29] Coselli JS, LeMaire SA, Köksoy C, Schmittling ZC, Curling PE. Cerebrospinal fluid drainage reduces paraplegia after thoracoabdominal aortic aneurysm repair: Results of a randomized clinical trial. Journal of Vascular Surgery. 2002;**35**(4):631–639

[30] Coselli JS, LeMaire SA, Orozco-Sevilla V, Preventza O, Moon MR, Barron LM, et al. Current approaches to spinal cord protection during open thoracoabdominal aortic aneurysm repair. Annals of Cardiothoracic Surgery 2023;**12**:429–437

[31] Trimarchi S, Tolenaar JL, Jonker FHW, Murray B, Tsai TT, Eagle KA, et al. Importance of false lumen thrombosis in type B aortic dissection prognosis. The Journal of Thoracic and Cardiovascular Surgery. 2013;**145**(3):S208–212

[32] Tolenaar JL, Eagle KA, Jonker FHW, Moll FL, Elefteriades JA, Trimarchi S. Partial thrombosis of the false lumen influences aortic growth in type B dissection. Annals of Cardiothoracic Surgery. 2014;**3**(3):275–277

[33] Tan SZCP, Jubouri M, Mohammed I, Bashir M. What is the long-term clinical efficacy of the thoraflex™ hybrid prosthesis for aortic arch repair? Frontiers in Cardiovascular Medicine. 2022;**9**:842165

[34] Kobuch R, Hilker M, Rupprecht L, Hirt S, Keyser A, Puehler T, et al. Late reoperations after repaired acute type A aortic dissection. The Journal of Thoracic and Cardiovascular Surgery 2012;**144**:300–307

[35] Pan E, Gudbjartsson T, Ahlsson A, Fuglsang S, Geirsson A, Hansson EC, et al. Low rate of reoperations after acute type A aortic dissection repair from The Nordic Consortium Registry. The Journal of Thoracic and Cardiovascular Surgery 2018;**156**: 939–948

[36] Iannelli G, Monaco M, Di Tommaso L, Piscione F. Complicated acute type B aortic dissection involving the arch: Treatment by simultaneous hybrid approach under local anesthesia. The Journal of Thoracic and Cardiovascular Surgery. 2008;**135**(6):1380–1382

[37] Coselli JS, Bozinovski J, LeMaire SA. Open surgical repair of 2286 thoracoabdominal aortic aneurysms. The Annals of Thoracic Surgery. discussion S890-892. 2007;**83** (2):S862–864

[38] Fujikawa T, Yamamoto S, Oshima S, Ozaki K, Shimamura J, Asada H, et al. Open surgery for descending thoracic aorta in an endovascular era. The Journal of Thoracic and Cardiovascular Surgery 2019;**157**:2168–2174

[39] Nienaber CA, Kische S, Rousseau H, Eggebrecht H, Rehders TC, Kundt G, et al. Endovascular repair of type B aortic dissection: Long-term results of the randomized investigation of stent grafts in aortic dissection trial. Circulation: Cardiovascular Interventions 2013;**6**:407–416

[40] Brunkwall J, Kasprzak P, Verhoeven E, Heijmen R, Taylor P, Trialists ADSORB, et al. Endovascular repair of acute uncomplicated aortic type B dissection promotes aortic remodelling: 1 year results of the ADSORB trial. European Journal of Vascular and Endovascular Surgery 2014;**48**:285–291

[41] Eggebrecht H, Thompson M, Rousseau H, Czerny M, Lönn L, Mehta RH, et al. Retrograde ascending aortic dissection during or after thoracic aortic stent graft placement: Insight from the European registry on endovascular aortic repair complications. Circulation. 2009;**120** (11_suppl_1):S276–281

[42] Rengel Z, Magee G. What can go wrong during thoracic endovascular aortic repair for type B aortic dissection. Journal of Vascular Surgery Cases, Innovations and Techniques. 2025;**11** (1):101657. Available from: https://www.jvscit.org/article/S2468-4287(24)00241-7/fulltext [cited 2025 Sept 9]

[43] Tsilimparis N, Detter C, Law Y, Rohlffs F, Heidemann F, Brickwedel J, et al. Single-center experience with an inner branched arch endograft. Journal of Vascular Surgery 2019;**69**:977–985.e1

[44] Ibrahim M, Lindsay TF, Chung JCY, Tan KT, Contreras J, Ouzounian M. Endovascular arch repair using the NEXUS arch endograft. Annals of Cardiothoracic Surgery. 2022;**11**(1):62–64

[45] Lella SK, Eagleton MJ, Sundt TM, Srivastava SD, Hosseini M, Bloom JP, et al. Feasibility of endovascular aortic arch repair after hemiarch replacement for acute type A aortic dissection. JTCVS Structural and Endovascular. 2024;**3**:100026

[46] Pang HJ, Warren AS, Dansey KD, Burke C, DeRoo S, Sweet MP, et al. Early outcomes of endovascular repairs of the aortic arch using thoracic branch endoprosthesis. Journal of Vascular Surgery 2024;**80**:22–31

[47] Nishina T, Yoshida Y, Mizuno A, Yada M, Yamanaka K. Is TEVAR with full petticoat technique effective for complicated acute type B dissection cases? Annals of Vascular Diseases. 2018;**11** (3):350–354

[48] Al-Rstum Z, Afifi RO. Retrograde aortic dissection during thoracic endovascular aortic repair: How to prevent and treat. jvascsurgc. 2024;**10**(4). Available from https://www.jvscit.org/article/S2468-4287(24)00108-4/fulltext [cited 2025 Sept 9]

[49] Bavaria J, Vallabhajosyula P, Moeller P, Szeto W, Desai N, Pochettino A. Hybrid approaches in the treatment of aortic arch aneurysms: Postoperative and midterm outcomes. The Journal of Thoracic and Cardiovascular Surgery. 2013;**145**(3):S85–90

[50] Nienaber CA, Rousseau H, Eggebrecht H, Kische S, Fattori R, Rehders TC, et al. Randomized comparison of strategies for type B aortic dissection: The INvestigation of STEnt Grafts in Aortic Dissection (INSTEAD) trial. Circulation 2009;**120**:2519–2528

[51] Kazimierczak A, Rynio P, Jędrzejczak T, Samad R, Rybicka A, Gutowski P. Aortic remodeling after extended PETTICOAT technique in acute aortic dissection type III B. Annals of Vascular Surgery. 2020;**66**:183–192

[52] Faure EM, El Batti S, Abou Rjeili M, Julia P, Alsac J-M. Mid-term outcomes of stent assisted balloon induced intimal disruption and relamination in aortic dissection repair (STABILISE) in acute type B aortic dissection. European Journal of Vascular and Endovascular Surgery. 2018;**56**(2):209–215

[53] Hofferberth SC, Nixon IK, Boston RC, McLachlan CS, Mossop PJ. Stent-assisted balloon-induced intimal disruption and relamination in Aortic dissection repair: The STABILISE concept. The Journal of Thoracic and Cardiovascular Surgery. 2014;**147** (4):1240–1245

[54] White A, Bozso SJ, Ouzounian M, Chu MWA, Moon MC. Acute type A aortic dissection and the consequences of a patent false lumen. JTCVS Techniques. 2021;**9**:1–8

[55] Crousillat D, Briller J, Aggarwal N, Cho L, Coutinho T, Harrington C, et al. Sex differences in thoracic aortic disease and dissection: JACC review topic of the week. Journal of the American College of Cardiology 2023;**82**:817–827

[56] Kölbel T, Carpenter SW, Lohrenz C, Tsilimparis N, Larena-Avellaneda A, Debus ES. Addressing persistent false lumen flow in chronic aortic dissection: The knickerbocker technique. Journal of Endovascular Therapy. 2014;**21**(1):117–122

[57] Tsai TT, Evangelista A, Nienaber CA, Trimarchi S, Sechtem U, Fattori R, et al. Long-term survival in patients presenting with type A acute aortic dissection: Insights from the International Registry of Acute Aortic Dissection (IRAD). Circulation 2006;**114**:I350–356

[58] Iglesias Iglesias C, González CC, Abril Ramiro F, Alonso Pastor A, Álvarez Marcos F, Alonso Pérez M. An early single-center experience with the Relay double inner-branch arch endograft. Journal of Thoracic Disease. 2023;**15**(12):6721–6729

[59] Murana G, Gliozzi G, Di Marco L, Campanini F, Snaidero S, Nocera C, et al. Frozen elephant trunk technique using hybrid grafts: 15-year outcomes from a single-centre experience. European Journal of Cardio-Thoracic Surgery. 2024;**65**(2):ezad364

[60] Etz CD, Kari FA, Mueller CS, Silovitz D, Brenner RM, Lin HM, et al. The collateral network concept: A reassessment of the anatomy of spinal cord perfusion. The Journal of Thoracic and Cardiovascular Surgery 2011;**141**:1020–1028

[61] Shimamura J, Abazid R, Gelinas J, Valdis M, Duncan A, Power A, et al. Five-year outcomes of hybrid arch frozen elephant trunk repair with novel multibranched hybrid graft. Annals of Thoracic Surgery Short Reports 2023;**1**:599–603

[62] Karangelis D, Stougiannou TM, Christodoulou KC, Bartolozzi H, Malafi ME, Mitropoulos F, et al. Hybrid aortic arch replacement with frozen elephant trunk (FET) technique: Surgical considerations, pearls, and pitfalls. Journal of Clinical Medicine 2024;**13**:7075

[63] Murana G, Campanini F, Orioli V, Pagano V, Santamaria V, Di Marco L,

et al. Frozen elephant trunk in acute aortic dissection: A literature review. Indian Journal of Thoracic and Cardiovascular Surgery. 2023;**39**(Suppl S2):315–324

[64] Shrestha M, Kaufeld T, Beckmann E, Fleissner F, Umminger J, Abd Alhadi F, et al. Total aortic arch replacement with a novel 4-branched frozen elephant trunk prosthesis: Single-center results of the first 100 patients. The Journal of Thoracic and Cardiovascular Surgery 2016;**152**: 148–159.e1

[65] Lawton JS, Liu J, Kulshrestha K, Moon MR, Damiano RJ, Maniar H, et al. The impact of surgical strategy on survival after repair of type A aortic dissection. The Journal of Thoracic and Cardiovascular Surgery 2015;**150**:294–301.e1

[66] Rong D, Ge Y, Liu J, Liu X, Guo W. Combined proximal descending aortic endografting plus distal bare metal stenting (PETTICOAT technique) versus conventional proximal descending aortic stent graft repair for complicated type B aortic dissections. The Cochrane Database of Systematic Reviews. 2019;**2019**(10):CD013149

Chapter 3

Aortic Root Surgery

Jakub Staromlynski and Piotr Suwalski

Abstract

The primary goal of minimally invasive surgery is to reduce perioperative trauma, accelerate patient mobilization, and shorten hospitalization time. Thanks to advances in modern technology, these procedures can now be offered to an increasingly broader group of patients. For many years, aortic root surgery was associated with the necessity of implanting a mechanical conduit, which required long-term anticoagulation therapy. Currently, in patients with an aortic root aneurysm and significant aortic regurgitation, valve-sparing reimplantation procedures can be performed via a minimally invasive approach. In the following chapter, we present a holistic description of the surgical technique for aortic root aneurysm repair using the reimplantation technique procedure while preserving the patient's native valve. We will focus on comprehensive imaging of the aorta prior to surgical intervention. This will allow us to present appropriate criteria for qualifying patients for the proposed surgical treatment, with particular emphasis on minimally invasive techniques. An essential part of the chapter will also include a detailed description of the entire procedure – starting from patient positioning on the operating table and the technique of chest opening, through the cannulation process for cardiopulmonary bypass, to a step-by-step explanation of the main procedure within the aortic root. The chapter will be rich in illustrations and photographs, making it a valuable resource for young cardiac surgeons, especially. It will provide a structured overview of minimally invasive cardiac surgery for aortic aneurysms, with a particular focus on aortic root surgery.

Keywords: aortic root surgery, aortic root reimplantation, aortic root replacement, minimally invasive approach, aorta imaging

1. Introduction

The number of diagnosed aortic aneurysms has been steadily increasing in recent years. This is strongly associated with the advancement of imaging techniques, as well as the broader availability of the most common noninvasive imaging modality for the heart and aorta – **transthoracic echocardiography (TTE)**. This trend is also related to the growing number of experienced echocardiographers, which enables the detection and close monitoring of aortic dilatations. As a result, patients can be qualified for surgical treatment at the appropriate time and under elective conditions. Such an approach improves surgical outcomes and reduces the risk of acute aortic dissection.

The development of medical technology has also driven the progress of **minimally invasive cardiac surgery**. Reducing the invasiveness of the procedure and minimizing the surgical access accelerates wound healing, functional recovery, and patient rehabilitation. Most importantly, this approach enhances the stability of the upper thoracic girdle, allowing patients to return earlier to full physical activity and professional life [1].

In the comprehensive qualification of a patient for surgical treatment of an aortic aneurysm, assessment by a **multidisciplinary "heart team"** is essential. Nowadays, due to the high degree of specialization and the complexity of treatment options, qualification should be performed within a dedicated **"aortic team."**

This team should include:

- A cardiac surgeon,
- A vascular surgeon,
- An interventional radiologist,
- An echocardiographer,
- And an anesthesiologist.

The role of this team is to conduct a thorough assessment of the indications, determine the extent of surgery, evaluate possible surgical approaches, and consider alternative or hybrid treatment strategies – particularly in high-risk patients in whom open surgery may be infeasible or when its risk outweighs the potential benefits [2].

2. Imaging of the aorta in qualification for surgical treatment

The most basic imaging modality in the initial assessment of the aorta is the chest X-ray. This examination may reveal a widened mediastinal shadow, which serves as an indication for further diagnostic imaging. However, the detection of mediastinal widening typically reflects an already advanced stage of aortic disease [3].

Patients with a confirmed significant aortic dilatation are referred for cardiothoracic surgical consultation (see **Figure 1**). In most cases, the initial finding of aortic enlargement is made using TTE. This test remains the fundamental tool for screening and preliminary evaluation, especially in the outpatient setting.

The advantages of TTE include its safety, repeatability, and broad availability. Nevertheless, it is considered a preliminary examination as it has limited value in intraoperative assessment.

During surgery, the imaging modality of choice is transesophageal echocardiography (TOE), which plays a crucial role in perioperative evaluation. TOE allows for detailed measurement of the aortic diameter at different levels, assessment of aortic valve morphology and function, as well as the dimensions and symmetry of the sinuses of Valsalva. It also enables differentiation between bicuspid (BAV) and tricuspid (TAV) aortic valve anatomy (see **Figure 2**) [4].

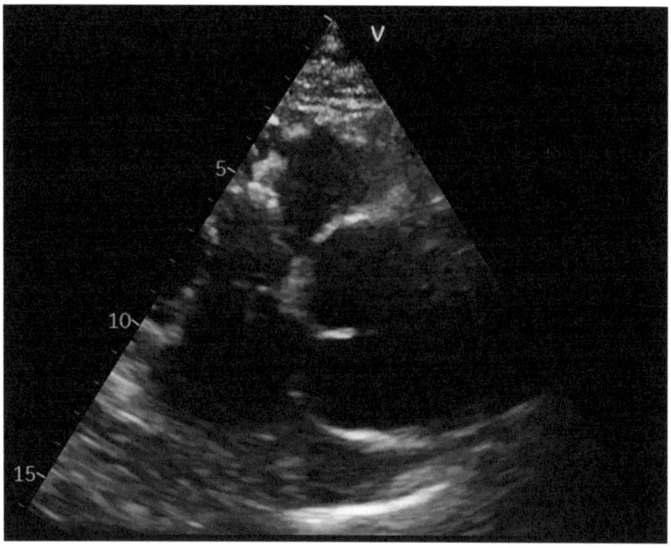

Figure 1.
Aortic root aneurysm in TTE.

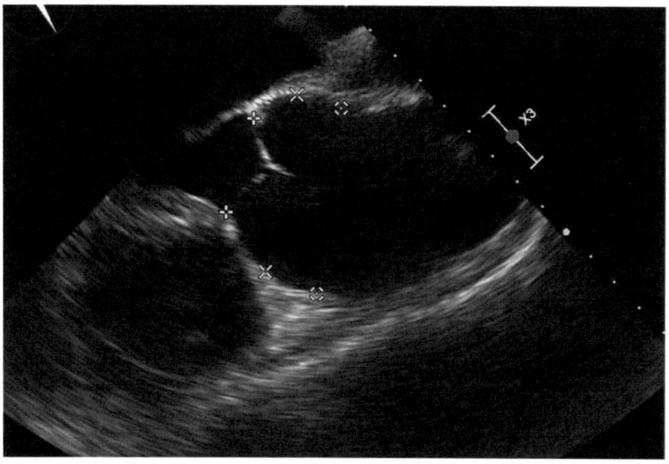

Figure 2.
Dimensions of the aorta based on TOE in root aneurysm.

In addition, TOE is used intraoperatively to verify the results of surgical correction during cardiac reperfusion, allowing immediate assessment of valve competence and the integrity of the repair (**Figure 3**).

Each patient undergoing qualification for cardiac surgery must have the diagnosis confirmed by computed tomography angiography (CTA). Both the European and American guidelines clearly recommend that this examination be performed with ECG gating in order to reduce the number of motion-related artifacts [5]. **Figure 4.**

CTA of the chest is not only used to confirm the diagnosis and assess the diameter of an aortic aneurysm, but it also provides other critical information essential for surgical planning. From a surgical standpoint, CTA is a key tool in preoperative

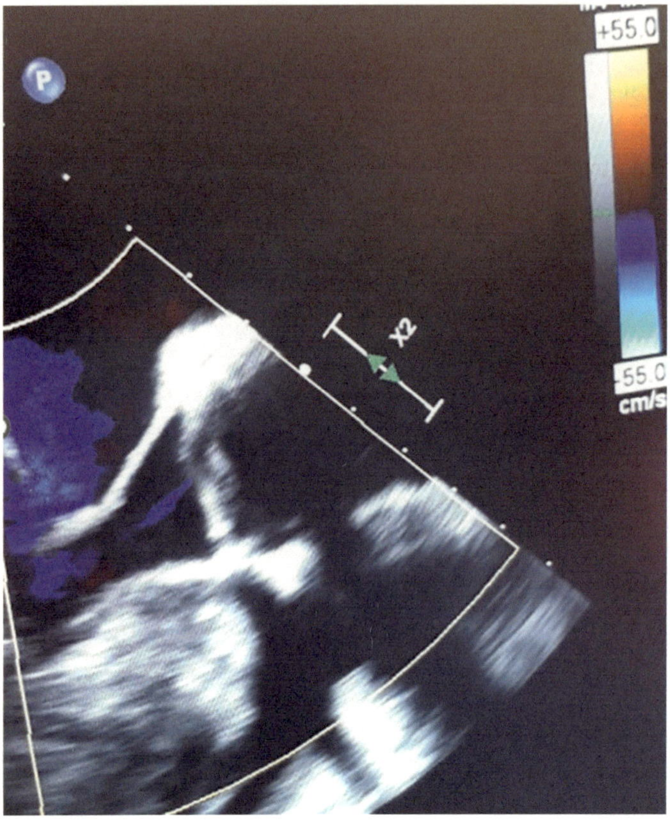

Figure 3.
Intraoperative TOE monitoring of aortic valve reimplantation using the David procedure.

assessment, as it allows for detailed evaluation of the position of the aorta within the mediastinum and its relationship to the sternum. This information is crucial for selecting the most appropriate operative approach.

The importance of this examination is particularly evident in minimally invasive procedures, such as partial upper ministernotomy or right anterior minithoracotomy (RAMT). The spatial orientation and distance of the aorta relative to the sternum play a decisive role in determining the optimal surgical access.

Three main configurations of the aortic position can be distinguished:

- Right-sided,
- Central, and
- Left-sided, relative to the sternum (see **Figure** 5).

Among these, the right-sided configuration is considered the most favorable, both for ministernotomy and minithoracotomy approaches. In this anatomical variant, the ascending aorta and its root are located closer to the operative field, facilitating exposure, dissection, and anastomotic suturing.

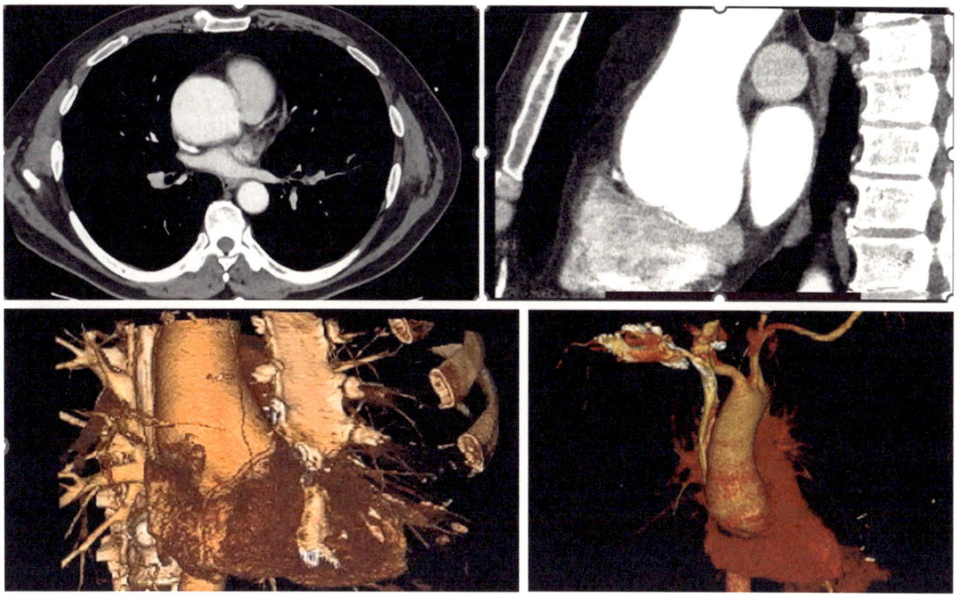

Figure 4.
Comprehensive assessment of the aortic root in chest CT angiography with ECG gating.

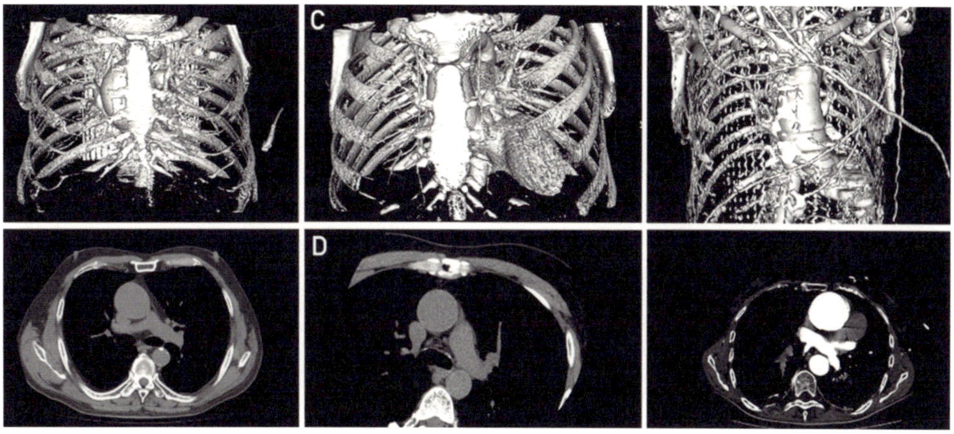

Figure 5.
Types of aortic positions relative to the breast bone in CT angiography.

Furthermore, CT imaging enables precise preoperative planning of the sternal incision, including its shape – J-, T-, or V-shaped – and the level of the intercostal space to be used (second, third, or fourth intercostal space) [6].

In many high-volume aortic centers, minimally invasive access has become the standard of care. The most experienced institutions have extended their expertise toward even less invasive approaches, such as RAMT or totally endoscopic access [7, 8].

In patients who cannot receive iodine-based contrast agents, magnetic resonance imaging (MRI) of the aorta with gadolinium administration remains a valuable alternative. This modality provides high-resolution and accurate imaging that is equally effective for assessing aortic morphology and for planning surgical treatment.

However, MRI is generally less accessible, the procedure is more time-consuming, and it requires strict patient cooperation to ensure diagnostic quality. Therefore, it is primarily reserved for a selected group of patients for whom CTA is contraindicated.

The most commonly used imaging modalities for aortic evaluation are compared in **Table 1**, while **Table 2** presents the recommended follow-up intervals based on the measured diameter of the aorta [9].

3. Indications for surgical treatment

Contemporary medicine allows for the qualification of patients for surgical treatment to be guided by evidence-based clinical criteria. The qualification standards are established and periodically updated by international scientific societies. Currently, the main sources of recommendations are the 2024 Guidelines of the European Association for Cardio-Thoracic Surgery (EACTS) and the

Imaging method	Clinical role	Advantages	Limitations	Follow-up/use
Chest X-ray	Initial, screening test	Quick, inexpensive	Low sensitivity and specificity	Not recommended for monitoring
CT angiography (CTA)	Gold standard – diagnosis and treatment planning	High spatial resolution, 3D reconstructions, rapid	Ionizing radiation, iodinated contrast	Follow-up every 6–12 months (based on diameter)
MR angiography (MRA)	Alternative to CT for long-term surveillance	No radiation, excellent soft-tissue, and flow detail	Longer scan, less availability	Preferred for genetic aortopathies/ repeated imaging
Transthoracic echocardiography (TTE)	Evaluation of ascending aorta	Noninvasive, widely available	Limited distal visualization	Initial evaluation, functional assessment
Transesophageal echocardiography (TOE)	Detailed evaluation of the ascending aorta and arch	High image quality, excellent in acute dissection	Semi-invasive, requires sedation	For unstable patients/suspected dissection
Conventional aortography	Primarily intraoperative (EVAR/ TEVAR)	Enables diagnosis and treatment together	Invasive, procedural risk	Not routinely used diagnostically

Table 1.
Comparison of aorta imaging methods according to the ESC 2024 guidelines.

Aneurysm diameter	Recommended interval (CT/MR)
<45 mm	Every 2–3 years
45–49 mm	Every 12 months
≥50 mm or growth >3 mm/year	Every 6 months
Postsurgery (TEVAR/open repair)	At 1, 6, and 12 months, then annually

Table 2.
Recommended imaging follow-up intervals according to ESC/ESVS 2022 guidelines.

European Society of Cardiology (ESC), as well as the 2022 Guidelines of the American College of Cardiology/American Heart Association (ACC/AHA) [4, 9].

A landmark study published by Parachuri et al. in 2015 has had a significant influence on the evolution of the indications for aortic aneurysm surgery over the past decade. The authors demonstrated a marked increase in the risk of aneurysm rupture when the aortic diameter exceeds 4.5 cm [9, 10].

In everyday clinical practice, it is essential to adhere to the recommendations issued by professional societies. These standardized criteria ensure a uniform and evidence-based approach to patient management in the majority of cases. Nevertheless, there remains a group of patients who do not fit conventional criteria and require individualized, multidisciplinary assessment, which improves procedural safety and overall outcomes.

3.1 Indications according to the 2024 ESC/EACTS guidelines

The 2024 ESC/EACTS guidelines on the management of thoracic aortic disease recommend surgical treatment in the following situations:

- Symptomatic thoracic aortic aneurysms, regardless of their diameter.
- Aneurysms with a maximal diameter ≥55 mm, irrespective of the presence of symptoms.
- Rapid expansion of the aneurysm, particularly if the diameter increases by >5 mm per year.
- Concomitant aortic valve disease, including regurgitation or stenosis.
- Aneurysms of the ascending aorta occur in patients with genetic syndromes such as Marfan syndrome or Ehlers–Danlos syndrome.
- Aneurysms of the ascending aorta in patients with bicuspid aortic valve (BAV), particularly when the diameter is ≥50 mm.
- In patients with TAV and low surgical risk, surgery may be considered at ≥52 mm in experienced centers (Class IIa recommendation).
- In patients undergoing concomitant aortic valve surgery, the threshold for aortic replacement may be lowered to ≥45–50 mm depending on the clinical context.

These guidelines emphasize the importance of individualized decision-making, taking into account the patient's age, general condition, comorbidities, anatomical characteristics, and personal preferences [9].

3.2 Indications according to the 2022 ACC/AHA guidelines

The 2022 ACC/AHA Guidelines for the Diagnosis and Management of Aortic Disease recommend surgical intervention in the following scenarios:

- Asymptomatic patients with aneurysms of the aortic root or ascending aorta when the maximal diameter is ≥5.5 cm (Class I recommendation).
- Aneurysms ≥50 mm in patients with genetic connective tissue disorders, such as Marfan or Ehlers–Danlos syndrome.
- Aneurysms ≥50 mm in patients with BAV.
- Aortic replacement during concomitant aortic valve surgery (surgical or TAVR) may be considered when the ascending aorta measures ≥4.5–5.0 cm, in centers with appropriate expertise.
- Aneurysm progression, defined as a diameter increase of ≥0.5 cm in one year or ≥0.3 cm/year over two consecutive years (for sporadic aneurysms), should prompt consideration of surgical repair.
- In patients with nonstandard body habitus (very tall, very short, or with low body surface area), the decision for surgery may be based on indexed aortic size (e.g., diameter-to-body surface area or diameter-to-height ratio).
- Symptomatic aneurysms, presenting with chest pain, dyspnea, or neurological symptoms, are also considered surgical indications.
- The presence of an ascending aortic aneurysm in patients with other cardiovascular diseases, such as coronary artery disease or heart failure, may also justify earlier surgical intervention.

Similar to the ESC recommendations, the AHA guidelines emphasize an individualized approach based on anatomical features, comorbidities, and patient preferences.

Furthermore, the guidelines highlight that aortic valve repair procedures (such as reimplantation or remodeling) – particularly when performed via minimally invasive approaches – should be undertaken only in high-volume centers with extensive experience in both valve-sparing aortic surgery and minimally invasive cardiac surgery (**Figure 6**) [4, 9].

4. Surgical approaches

From the cardiac surgeon's perspective, the choice of surgical access is of paramount importance for the safe and effective performance of an aortic operation. The primary objective in surgical planning must always be patient safety. Not every patient is an appropriate candidate for a minimally invasive procedure. The choice of approach depends on the patient's anatomy, history of prior thoracic surgeries, and particularly the position of the aorta within the mediastinum.

During the qualification process, the following factors must be carefully evaluated:

- The patient's preferences and expectations,

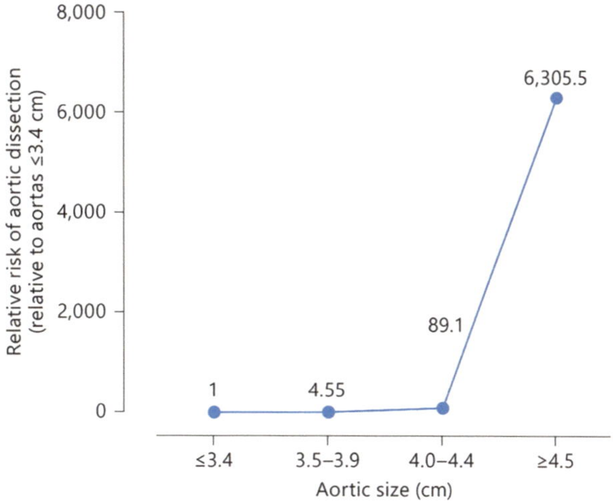

Figure 6.
Relative risk of aortic dissection by size range, based on the 2022 ACC/AHA guideline for the diagnosis and management of aortic disease.

- The anatomical characteristics of the aorta (its position and depth within the mediastinum),
- Thoracic anatomy (including congenital chest wall deformities such as pectus carinatum or pectus excavatum),
- The availability of equipment (endoscope, minimally invasive instruments, soft tissue retractors),
- The experience of the anesthesiology and surgical team, and
- The institutional experience in performing minimally invasive aortic surgery.

4.1 Contraindications and limiting factors for minimally invasive access

Certain anatomical or clinical features may limit or contraindicate a minimally invasive approach, including:

- Unfavorable chest wall anatomy (pectus carinatum or pectus excavatum),
- Large or complex aneurysms (some studies suggest that an aneurysm diameter >67 mm constitutes a contraindication due to restricted visual field, difficulties in safe clamping, and risk of uncontrolled bleeding) (**Figure** 7) [11],
- Acute aortic dissection,

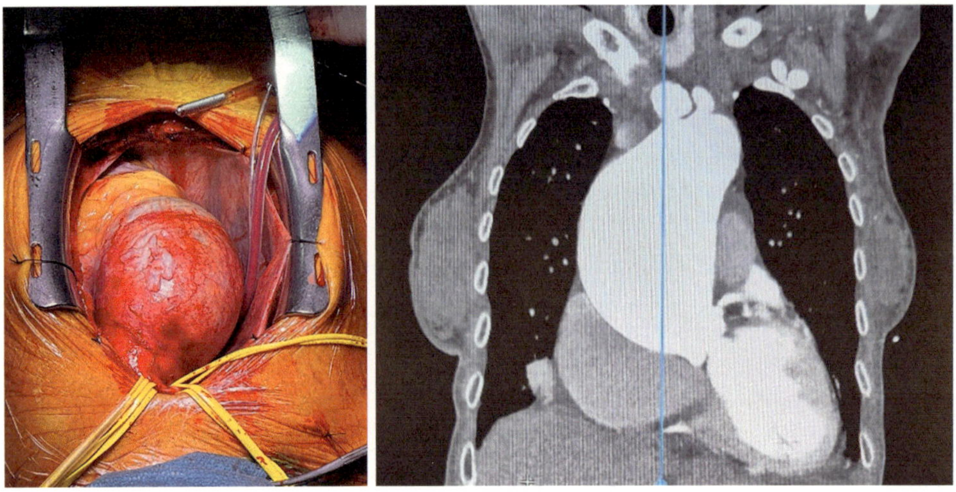

Figure 7.
Complex giant aneurysm: surgical view and preoperative CTA.

- Reoperations or previous thoracic procedures with dense adhesions,
- Respiratory insufficiency ($FEV_1 < 40\%$), since one-lung ventilation required for minithoracotomy or thoracoscopic procedures can worsen respiratory function and increase pulmonary complications,
- Inability to perform safe peripheral cannulation, and
- Active infection at the surgical site [12].

4.2 Technological advancements

Modern surgical technology has significantly facilitated the reduction of surgical access through the use of high-definition endoscopic visualization. In leading centers, 3D thoracoscopic systems with 4K resolution have become the standard of care, enabling high precision and superior depth perception [13].

4.3 Types of surgical access

The planning of an aortic procedure should always begin with the selection of the surgical approach. In contemporary cardiac surgery, aside from the standard full median sternotomy, various partial sternotomy techniques are available, including:

- J-shaped sternotomy (extending into the right or left intercostal space),
- T-shaped sternotomy, and
- V-shaped sternotomy.

The choice of access depends on several factors, but the two most critical are:

- The surgeon's experience, and
- The patient's anatomical conditions.

Figure 8. Illustrates several examples of minimally invasive approaches to the thoracic aorta

4.4 Partial sternotomy approaches

Currently, the J-shaped upper ministernotomy, performed through the third intercostal space and extending toward the right pleural cavity, is the most widely adopted approach. Some surgeons advocate extending the incision toward the left side, which may improve exposure and operator comfort. However, current evidence does not clearly support the superiority of either direction [14].

The V-shaped ministernotomy provides the widest exposure to both the aortic root and the proximal aortic arch, making it a reasonable option for surgeons at the beginning of their experience with minimally invasive aortic procedures. Its potential drawback is partial sternal instability, which, in rare cases, may require refixation. Nevertheless, proper sternal closure at the time of the primary operation effectively prevents this complication [15].

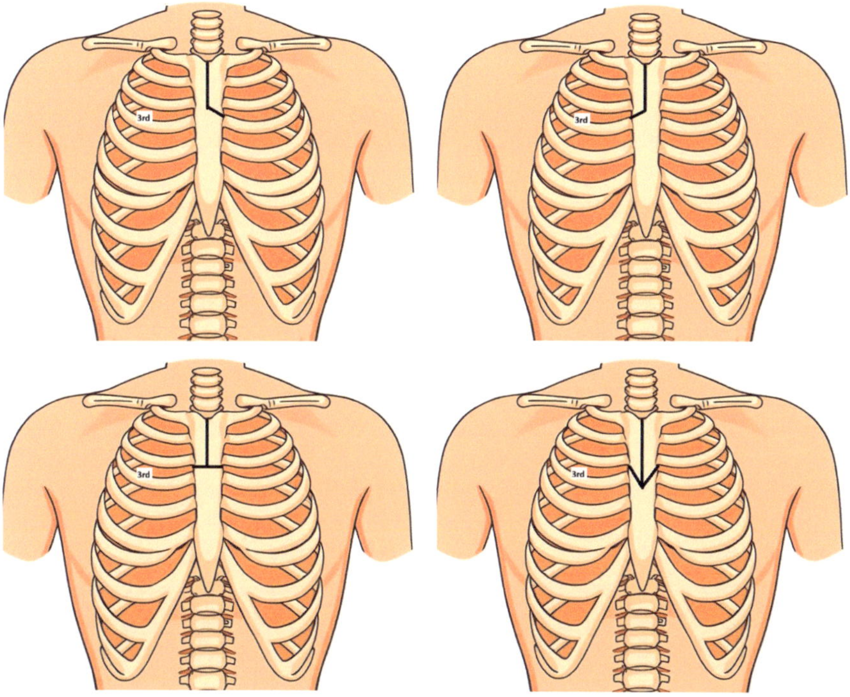

Figure 8.
Different types of partial ministernotomy (J both sides, t and V-shape). The illustration was created with the use of AI tools.

The J-shaped ministernotomy is considered the least invasive approach, causing minimal disruption to the thoracic and shoulder girdle integrity. It has been shown to reduce the risk of sternal bleeding, shorten postoperative mobilization time, decrease respiratory complications, and accelerate rehabilitation and recovery [15, 16].

The transverse sternal division can be made either at the third or fourth intercostal space, depending on the anatomy and depth of the ascending aorta within the mediastinum [17].

4.5 Right anterior minithoracotomy (RAMT) and transaxillary (TAX) approaches

Recent reports have described successful, complex aortic root operations performed through RAMT or even totally endoscopic transaxillary (TAX) approaches. These techniques require a high level of surgical skill and careful patient selection based on anatomical suitability.

The advantages for the patient include:

- Reduced surgical trauma,
- Lower intraoperative blood loss (due to avoidance of sternal division),
- Shorter hospital stay, and
- Superior cosmetic results.

This cosmetic advantage is especially relevant in young female patients, as the incision can be placed within the natural inframammary fold along the lateral chest wall.

However, large comparative trials are still lacking, and current evidence is based mainly on single-center studies or case reports of aortic root surgery performed via minithoracotomy or endoscopic access [18]. With the continuous development of endoscopic and robotic technology, these approaches are expected to become increasingly widespread in the near future.

4.6 Technical considerations in minithoracotomy

When performing a minithoracotomy, the choice of intercostal space for the main working port is critical – most often the third or fourth, and less frequently the second intercostal space. The endoscopic camera is typically inserted through the second intercostal space in the anterior axillary line, while the aortic cross-clamp is introduced via a separate incision in the second intercostal space along the midaxillary line.

Depending on the surgeon's preference, flexible or bead-type cross-clamps may be used and can even be introduced directly through the main working incision (**Figures 9** and **10**).

Thoracoscopy plays a central role in these minimally invasive operations. In most cases, cardiopulmonary bypass is established via peripheral cannulation – using the femoral or subclavian artery and femoral vein. In selected patients, if the anatomy permits, central cannulation of the ascending aorta and right atrium may also be performed [18].

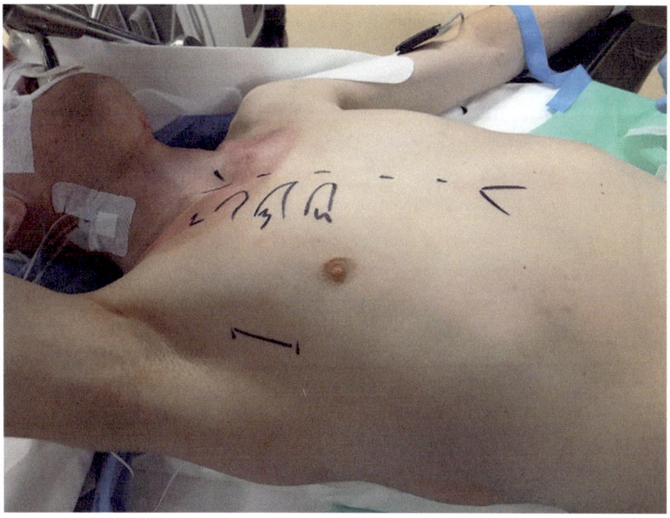

Figure 9.
Skin incision: TAX approach.

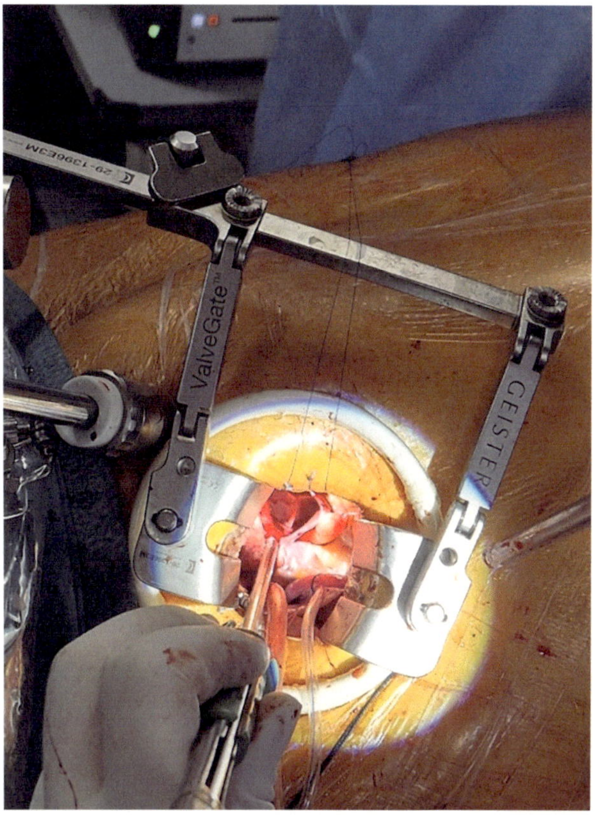

Figure 10.
Axillary access (TAX): replacement of the aortic valve and ascending aorta.

5. Cannulation techniques

In minimally invasive cardiac surgery, the technique of cannulation and extracorporeal circulation management plays a crucial role.

In procedures performed through partial upper ministernotomy, direct cannulation of the ascending aorta and the right atrium is possible [14]. The aortic cannula may be inserted high, at the level of the proximal aortic arch, which allows placement of the cross-clamp in a correspondingly high position. The right atrium can be cannulated using a two-stage or three-stage venous cannula.

It is advisable to pass the venous cannula beneath the sternum and exteriorize it through a small subxiphoid incision. This technique creates additional space within the mediastinum, thereby bringing the aortic root closer to the operative field and improving exposure (**Figure 11**).

5.1 Peripheral cannulation in minithoracotomy

In RAMT approaches, peripheral cannulation is the preferred method. The right femoral vessels (artery and vein) in the groin are most commonly used, while the right subclavian artery may serve as an alternative arterial site.

In recent years, percutaneous cannulation techniques have become increasingly popular and are often preferred over open surgical exposure (**Figure 12**).

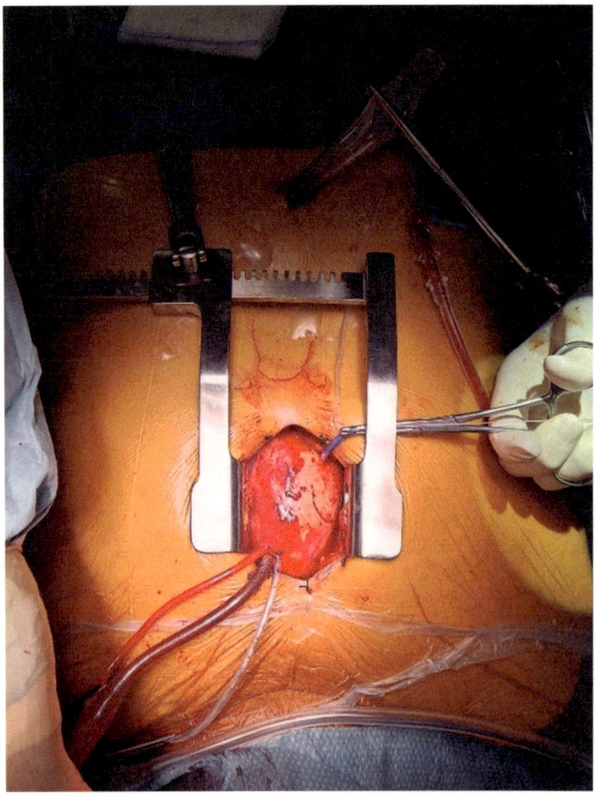

Figure 11.
Technique of central cannulation via J-ministernotomy.

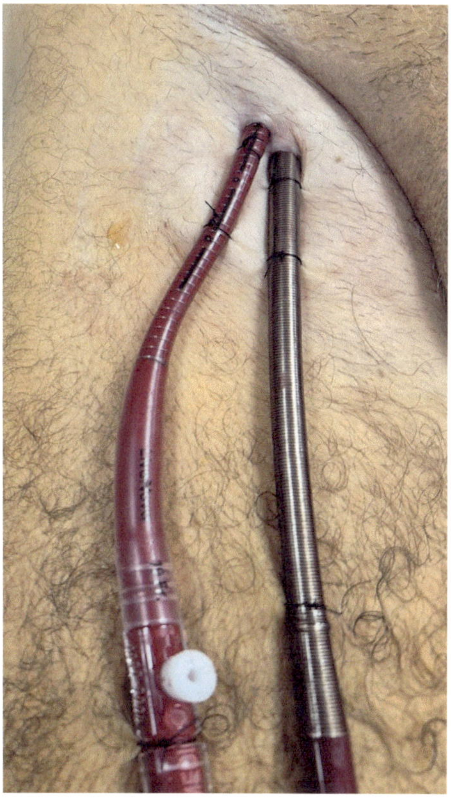

Figure 12.
Percutaneous right groin cannulation.

Cannulation is typically performed using the Seldinger technique under ultrasound (USG) guidance.

The position of the guidewire in the superior vena cava and descending aorta should be verified intraoperatively by TOE [19].

5.2 Advantages and risks of peripheral cannulation

Peripheral cannulation offers numerous advantages, including improved surgical exposure and the ability to maintain a limited operative field. However, this technique is also associated with several potential complications, such as:

- Retrograde dissection of the thoracic aorta,
- Local arterial or venous injury at the puncture site,
- Retroperitoneal hematoma,
- Pseudoaneurysm,

- Chylous leakage, and
- Groin wound infection.

To minimize these risks, USG and TOE guidance should always be used during the procedure. In many cases, effective venous drainage requires the application of negative pressure on the venous line to maintain adequate flow [22].

A summary of the advantages and limitations of peripheral cannulation is presented in **Table 3** [20, 21].

5.3 Venting techniques

In both direct and peripheral cannulation setups, left heart venting is typically performed through the right superior pulmonary vein, with the cannula positioned into the left ventricle under TOE guidance. This approach ensures effective left ventricular decompression and facilitates controlled cardiac reperfusion [20, 21].

6. Surgical techniques

Aortic root surgery represents one of the most technically demanding and advanced areas of cardiac surgery. Procedures in this region are primarily indicated in cases of ascending aortic aneurysm involving the aortic annulus, congenital aortic dilatation (e.g., Marfan, Loeys–Dietz, or Ehlers–Danlos syndromes), and complex aortic valve pathologies associated with dilatation of the sinuses of Valsalva. The goal

Aspect	Peripheral cannulation	Central cannulation
Perfusion direction	Femoral = retrograde; Axillary = antegrade	Antegrade (direct aortic cannulation)
Stroke/embolic risk	Higher with femoral (retrograde → risk of atheroembolism); lower with axillary	Lower if the ascending aorta is disease-free; risk increases with manipulation in an atherosclerotic aorta
Local vascular complications	Hematoma, pseudoaneurysm, wound infection, limb ischemia	Local bleeding at the operative site, rarely distal ischemic complications
Risk of adjacent structure injury	Axillary – possible brachial plexus injury; Femoral – possible femoral nerve injury	Possible injury to the aorta or atrial wall during manipulation
CPB initiation (before chest opening)	Feasible externally – a major advantage in high-risk aneurysms	Usually only possible after sternotomy and exposure
Venous drainage efficiency	May require dual venous cannulas or vacuum-assisted drainage	Standard and effective in most cases
Main limitations	Atherosclerotic or stenotic peripheral vessels; limb ischemia risk (femoral)	Limited exposure in MICS; manipulation risk on a fragile aorta

Table 3.
Comparison – peripheral versus central cannulation for cardiopulmonary bypass in minimally invasive aortic surgery.

of surgery is not only to excise the diseased segment of the aortic wall but also to restore the normal geometry of the aortic root and valve apparatus, ensuring durable hemodynamic function of the native valve.

Currently, three main operative techniques are available for addressing complex aortic root pathology:

- Bentall–De Bono procedure – composite aortic root replacement,
- David procedure – valve-sparing root reimplantation,
- Yacoub procedure – remodeling of the aortic root, an alternative valve-sparing approach that recreates the anatomy of the sinuses of Valsalva without fully reimplanting the valve annulus.

Each of these techniques has its own specific indications, advantages, and limitations, and the choice of procedure depends on the root morphology, valve condition, comorbidities, and experience of the surgical center.

6.1 Valve-sparing root reimplantation – the David procedure

One of the most frequently performed operations for aortic root aneurysm with significant aortic regurgitation is the valve-sparing aortic root reimplantation, first described by Tirone David [22]. The key elements of this procedure include excision of the aneurysmal sinuses, restoration of cusp coaptation, and stabilization of the aortic annulus. This is achieved by excising the sinuses of Valsalva, constructing a new aortic root using a vascular graft, and reimplanting the aortic valve commissures at their appropriate height.

Two critical steps in this operation are:

- Selecting the correct size of the vascular graft, and
- Determining the proper height of commissural suspension to ensure optimal cusp coaptation.

After cardioplegic arrest, the ascending aorta is transected at the level of the sinotubular junction (STJ). The surgeon then assesses the number and morphology of the cusps, as well as the coronary ostia, including their location and course – these steps are essential for the success of the procedure.

Using the Schäfer's caliper and a ruler, both geometric height (Gh) and effective height (Eh) of the cusps are measured:

- Geometric height (Gh): measured from the cusp insertion line to the free margin. In adults, this is typically 17–21 mm; a value of ≥18 mm qualifies the valve for reimplantation. In BAV, the Gh should be ≥19–21 mm.
- Effective height (Eh): measured from the aortic annular plane (above the LVOT) to the coaptation point of the cusp when filled with saline. This should measure ≥9 mm, as determined with the Schäfer's caliper [23].

The aortic annulus diameter is then measured using Hegar dilators or a spherical sizer, typically ranging from 23 to 27 mm. The graft diameter is usually selected to be 4–6 mm larger than the annulus. In BAV cases, a graft only 2 mm larger is generally chosen, as the annulus is already dilated and cusp geometry is asymmetric. Cusp plication or, less commonly, patch augmentation using autologous pericardium may be required [24].

Once all measurements confirm suitability for reimplantation, the coronary ostia are excised as buttons, the dilated sinuses are resected, and the aortic root is dissected free from surrounding tissues, leaving a 5–6 mm rim of native aortic wall to be sutured into the graft (**Figure 13**).

6.2 Annular stabilization

Annular stabilization is a critical step in the procedure, and several techniques have been described – external, internal, or subcommissural. Although there is no universal consensus, most surgeons agree that annular stabilization is essential. Typically, 12–14 pledgeted horizontal mattress sutures are placed circumferentially around the native annulus, starting from the left ventricular outflow tract (LVOT). One suture is placed at each commissure and three between commissures (**Figure 14**).

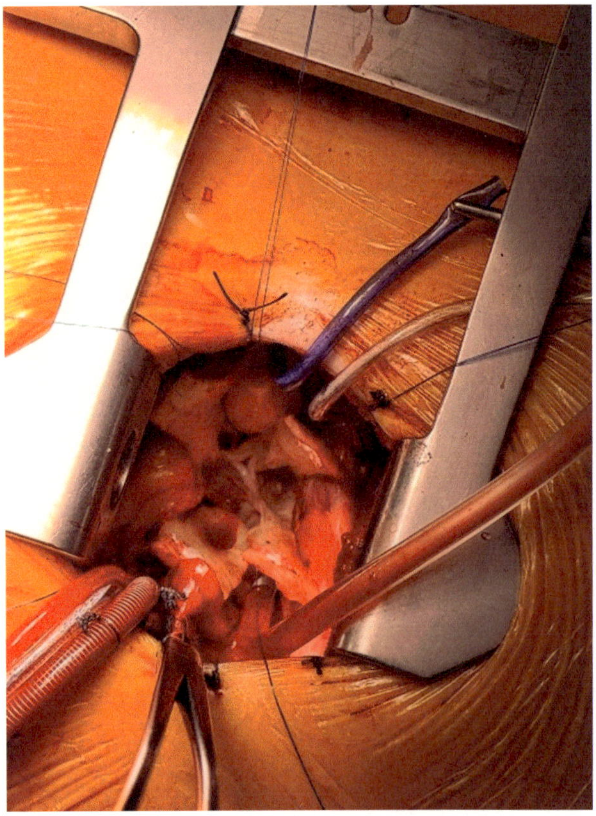

Figure 13.
Aortic root ready for aortic reimplantation.

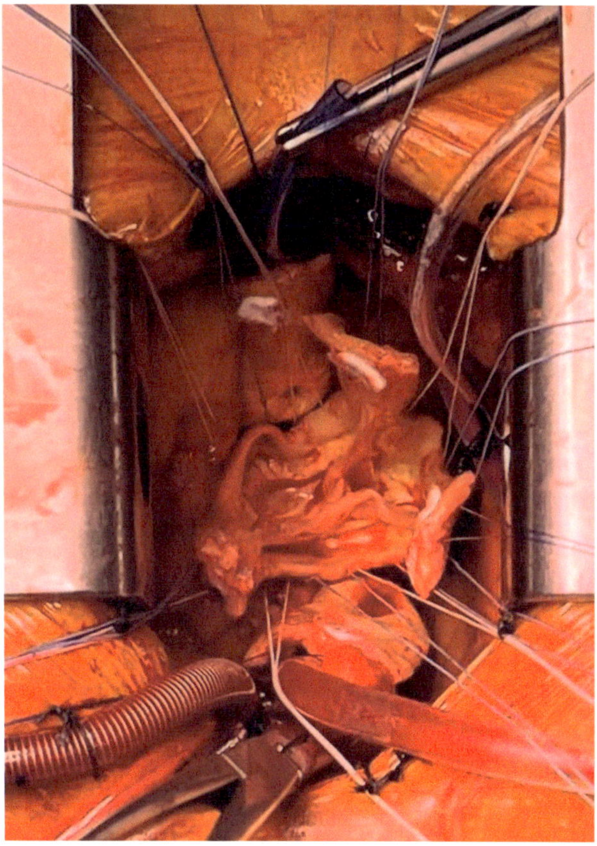

Figure 14.
Aortic root stabilization with pledget sutures: J-ministernotomy approach.

Special caution must be exercised near the right–noncoronary commissure, as the conduction system runs close to the base of this area. To avoid postoperative heart block, sutures should be placed strictly at the apex of the intercommissural triangle [25–27].

6.3 Graft implantation and commissural reimplantation

After annular sutures are placed, the graft is anchored to the annulus, and the commissures are reimplanted at the predetermined height. A frequently discussed topic concerns the choice between a straight graft and a Valsalva graft.

The Valsalva graft offers potentially better hemodynamic performance, improved cusp motion, and enhanced coronary flow due to its sinus geometry. Conversely, the straight graft provides simpler sizing and predictable geometry, with comparable long-term durability, according to several studies [28]. There is no conclusive evidence favoring one graft type over the other; however, many centers, including ours, routinely use straight tubular grafts without sinuses.

To facilitate commissural alignment, the new commissure positions may be marked on the graft with a sterile marker. When tying the annular sutures, care must be taken to avoid narrowing the LVOT; a Hegar dilator can be temporarily inserted through the annulus to maintain lumen patency.

The native aortic wall remnants are then sutured to the inner surface of the graft using a continuous 4–0 or 5–0 polypropylene suture, depending on tissue quality and surgeon preference, thereby creating a neo-root or neo-aorta.

At this stage, a final measurement of cusp coaptation height is performed and should range between 8 and 10 mm [28, 29].

6.4 Coronary reimplantation and distal anastomosis

In the final stages, both coronary buttons are reimplanted into the graft (**Figure 15**). The distal graft anastomosis is then completed to the proximal aortic arch using 5–0 polypropylene suture (**Figure 16**).

Following rewarming and reperfusion, intraoperative TOE is performed to assess valve competence. The goal is a competent aortic valve with proper cusp coaptation (trace or mild regurgitation acceptable) and a transvalvular gradient < 10 mmHg [30].

A representative video of the procedure is available in *Video 1 (URL: ...)*.

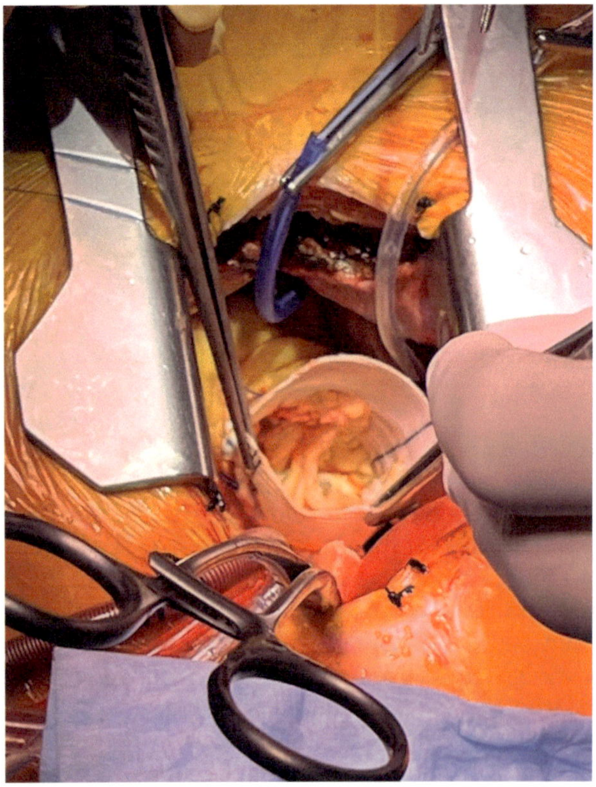

Figure 15.
Complete aortic root reimplantation: J-ministernotomy approach.

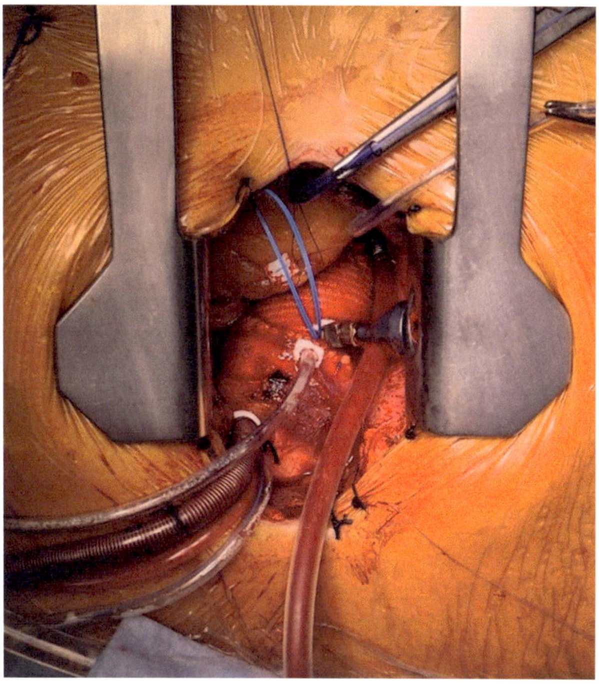

Figure 16.
Final view of David procedure via J-ministernotomy approach.

6.5 Summary

The David valve-sparing reimplantation procedure is now an established and effective surgical method for treating aortic root aneurysms in patients with preserved cusp morphology. By preserving the native aortic valve and restoring the anatomical geometry of the aortic root, this technique provides excellent hemodynamic outcomes while eliminating the need for lifelong anticoagulation therapy.

6.6 Bentall–De Bono procedure

The Bentall–De Bono procedure is indicated when there are clear indications for the replacement of both the aortic valve and the aortic root. Typical indications include:

- Aortic root aneurysm requiring concomitant aortic valve replacement,
- Aortic root dissection, not suitable for valve-sparing repair, is often associated with connective tissue disorders such as Marfan or Loeys–Dietz syndrome,
- Infective endocarditis with annular destruction, and
- Secondary aortic root dilation following previous aortic valve replacement.

After cardioplegic arrest, the aorta is transected just above the STJ. The valve and root are inspected to confirm the indication for root replacement. The coronary ostia are carefully evaluated – their number, location, and initial course – as these features are crucial for safe mobilization and reimplantation, helping to prevent complications such as kinking or coronary malperfusion [31].

Following coronary mobilization, the native aortic valve is excised, and decannulation and debridement of the annulus are performed to prepare the site for implantation. Pledgeted sutures are commonly used to secure the conduit to the annulus.

6.6.1 Intraannular versus supra-annular (inverted) implantation

The valved conduit can be implanted either intraannularly or supra-annularly. Accurate sizing of the aortic annulus and careful graft selection are critical to avoid oversizing, which could damage the native annulus and result in catastrophic bleeding.

The choice between intra- and supra-annular (inverted) implantation techniques remains a subject of debate. Some studies suggest that supra-annular (inverted) implantation reduces the overall conduit size, likely due to the annular stiffening effect of pledgets. Conversely, the supra-annular position may better replicate the anatomical alignment and provide improved hemodynamic performance (**Figure 17**).

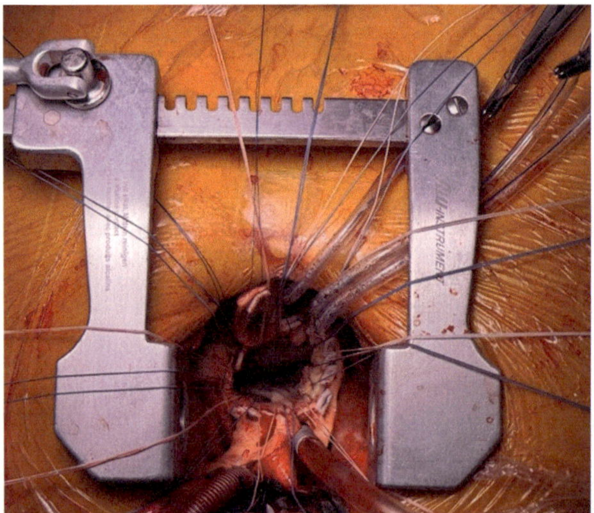

Figure 17.
Suprannular implantation technique with inverted, patch-reinforced sutures in the invasive Bentall de Bono procedure.

Intraannular implantation, on the other hand, may be particularly advantageous in patients with small annuli or endocarditis, where the tissues are fragile and nondistensible [32, 33]. Although no definitive studies confirm the superiority of either method, some authors report that the inverted supra-annular technique offers better postoperative hemostasis in the root area [34].

6.6.2 Choice of conduit – mechanical versus biological

A crucial decision during the Bentall procedure is the choice of valved conduit – mechanical or biological. This decision should be individualized, taking into account:

- Patient preferences and lifestyle,
- Age,
- Potential desire for pregnancy (in younger women),
- Risk of bleeding or thrombosis, and
- Contraindications to long-term anticoagulation.

In most reports, mechanical conduits demonstrate superior long-term durability [35, 36]. However, in patients over 65 years of age or those with contraindications to lifelong anticoagulation, a biological conduit remains the preferred option. In the event of structural valve degeneration, a transcatheter valve-in-valve (TAVR–ViV) procedure can be considered as a secondary intervention [37].

6.6.3 Prefabricated and custom-made conduits

Both mechanical and biological prefabricated conduits are currently available. In 2025, a new biological valved conduit – Konect – was introduced, incorporating the Inspiris Resilia aortic valve (Edwards Lifesciences, Irvine, CA, USA) [38]. This prosthesis utilizes glycerolization and aldehyde stabilization technology, which reduces calcium deposition and delays structural valve degeneration – effects that have been confirmed in in vitro testing [39]. The implantation technique for this prosthesis is illustrated in **Figure 18**.

When a suitable prefabricated conduit is not available, the surgeon may construct a custom-made aortic conduit using any combination of an aortic prosthetic graft and a separate aortic valve prosthesis. The diameter of the chosen graft is typically 5 mm larger than the valve size to ensure proper alignment. The two components are joined using a continuous 4–0 or 5–0 polypropylene suture [36–39]. The assembly technique is shown in **Figure 19**.

An additional hemostatic modification, known as the "French cuff" technique, involves retaining a short collar of the vascular graft when attaching the prosthetic valve to the conduit. This cuff improves hemostasis and facilitates potential future reoperations, as it enables valve replacement without disrupting the graft or requiring coronary reimplantation [40].

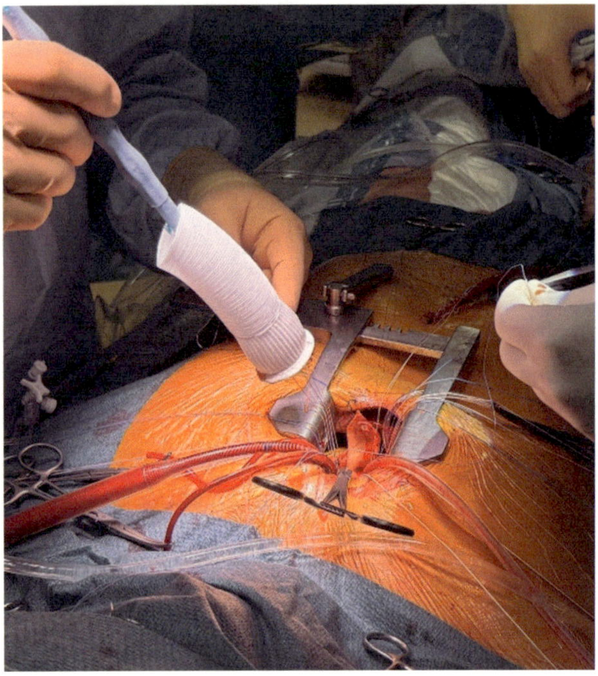

Figure 18.
KONECT INSPIRIS RESILIA conduit implantation (Edwards Lifesciences, Irvine, CA, USA).

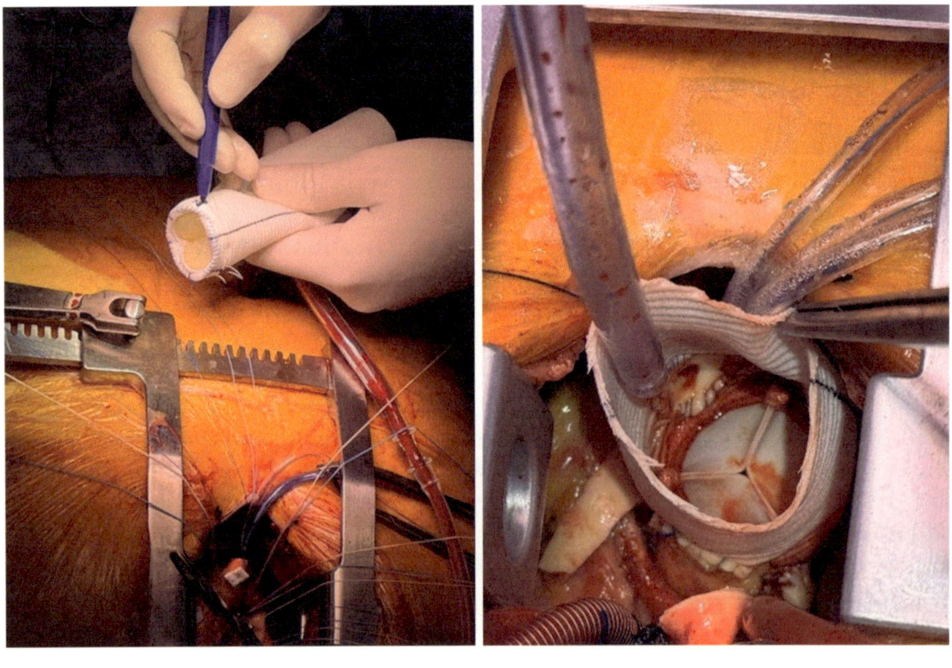

Figure 19.
Manual construction of a composite graft using an Inspiris Resilia bioprosthetic valve (Edwards Lifesciences, Irvine, CA, USA) and a Hemashield Platinum woven graft (Maquet Getinge Group, Rastatt, Germany).

6.6.4 Completion of the procedure

After the preparation of the conduit, the next steps include the reimplantation of the coronary buttons and the construction of the distal anastomosis.

The Bentall–De Bono procedure remains the gold standard for the management of aortic root aneurysms and pathologies involving the aortic valve and root. Over time, the evolution of the technique – from Hugh Bentall's original description to modern modifications incorporating prefabricated conduits and advanced bioprosthetic valves – has significantly improved surgical safety and long-term outcomes.

The choice between a mechanical or biological conduit, and between intra- or supra-annular implantation (with or without hemostatic modifications, such as the French cuff technique), should always be individualized based on patient age, risk profile, and expected life expectancy.

6.7 Root remodeling

The Yacoub aortic root remodeling procedure is a valve-sparing operation performed on patients with an aortic root aneurysm and preserved aortic valve morphology. The technique involves the resection of the dilated sinuses of Valsalva and their replacement with a tailored Dacron graft, shaped to reproduce the three sinuses and restore the physiological geometry of the aortic root. The native aortic valve remains in situ, while the coronary arteries are reimplanted into the new graft.

Indications:

- Aortic root aneurysm with intact or minimally diseased aortic cusps,
- Connective tissue disorders (e.g., Marfan syndrome) with adequate cusp quality,
- Younger patients in whom lifelong anticoagulation is undesirable.

Contraindications:

- Significant cusp degeneration or calcification,
- Advanced aortic regurgitation with cusp distortion,
- Severe annular dilatation or structural damage, precluding secure fixation.

The Yacoub remodeling technique enables preservation of the native aortic valve and restoration of normal aortic root dynamics. However, compared with the David reimplantation technique, it carries a higher risk of late aortic regurgitation, as the aortic annulus is not fixed within the graft. Therefore, the choice between Yacoub and David procedures depends on the anatomy of the root and the degree of annular dilatation [41, 42].

As always, there are supporters and opponents of the method. The Yacoub operation (remodeling) is an excellent technique for patients with a well-preserved aortic valve and a stable annulus, particularly in young individuals without connective tissue disease. It allows preservation of the native valve, natural hemodynamics, and avoidance of anticoagulation.

However, due to the risk of late aortic regurgitation and the lack of annular stabilization, in cases of annular dilation or connective tissue disease, the David operation is preferred today [43].

6.8 Ross procedure – use of homografts and xenografts

The Ross procedure, which involves the autograft replacement of the aortic valve using the patient's pulmonary valve and the substitution of the pulmonary position with a homograft or xenograft, was first introduced in 1967 for the surgical treatment of aortic root disease. This technique allows for the restoration of physiological aortic valve function, excellent hemodynamics, and the elimination of lifelong anticoagulation therapy.

However, the operation is contraindicated in patients with a markedly dilated aortic annulus or those with abnormal pulmonary valve morphology. Despite these limitations, the Ross procedure is currently experiencing a renaissance in many specialized centers worldwide.

6.8.1 Surgical technique

The pulmonary autograft is harvested to include the pulmonary valve along with 3–5 mm of adjacent right ventricular muscle at its base. The autograft can be implanted using one of two techniques:

- Full-root replacement – following the complete excision of the aortic valve and the sinuses of Valsalva, or

- Subcoronary implantation – preserving the native aortic sinuses.

The graft is sutured using a continuous 4–0 or 5–0 polypropylene suture. In some cases, the aortic annulus may require reinforcement with a Teflon strip to prevent postoperative dilatation. In the pulmonary position, either a homograft or a xenograft is implanted to restore right ventricular outflow tract (RVOT) continuity.

6.8.2 Xenografts

One limitation of the Ross operation is the limited availability of homografts from tissue banks, which often necessitates the use of xenografts as an alternative. The most commonly used xenografts include:

- Contegra® (Medtronic, Minneapolis, MN, USA),

- BioValsalva® (Vascutek Terumo, Renfrewshire, Scotland, UK),

- Freestyle® (Medtronic Inc., Minneapolis, USA).

A xenograft is a biological prosthesis made from animal tissue (most commonly bovine pericardium or porcine aortic valve tissue), either integrated into a synthetic vascular graft or prefabricated as a complete valved conduit.

The main advantages of xenografts are:

- Excellent hemodynamic performance,
- Wide availability, and
- Ease of implementation.

However, their disadvantages include:

- Limited durability, and
- Risk of premature structural valve degeneration.

The choice of a specific xenograft depends on several factors, including patient age, tissue availability, institutional experience, and the expected lifespan of the graft [37–43].

6.8.3 Homografts

A homograft (or allograft) consists of a human aortic valve with an attached segment of the ascending aorta, harvested from a human donor, preserved, and stored under cryogenic conditions. Homografts are used for total aortic root replacement (full-root replacement) or as an aortic valve substitute in reconstructive procedures.

Currently, the main indications for homograft use include:

- Infective endocarditis with annular destruction,
- Disruption of the mitral–aortic continuity with abscess or fistula formation, and
- Redo operations involving the aortic root.

The primary advantage of homografts lies in the low susceptibility of human tissue to bacterial colonization compared to synthetic or animal-derived materials, as well as their near-physiologic hemodynamic performance.

Their main limitations are the limited availability in tissue banks and the restricted range of available sizes.

From a technical standpoint, the most commonly used method is the full-root replacement technique, with coronary buttons reimplanted directly into the homograft wall. Additionally, homografts can be used as patch material for reconstruction of the LVOT in cases of extensive abscess formation with destruction of the surrounding tissues [44, 45].

6.8.4 Summary

The Ross procedure, through the use of pulmonary autografts combined with homograft or xenograft replacement of the pulmonary position, offers physiological aortic valve function, excellent hemodynamic results, and freedom from anticoagulation. Although technically demanding and limited by tissue availability, this operation remains a valuable option for selected patients, especially young adults and children, providing durable results when performed in experienced centers.

7. Overview

Aortic root surgery remains the gold standard in the surgical management of complex aortic aneurysms and aortic valve diseases. The choice of technique depends on the patient's anatomy, age, and individual preference.

The David procedure (valve-sparing root reimplantation) preserves the patient's native valve and provides excellent long-term outcomes without the need for lifelong anticoagulation. However, it requires considerable surgical expertise, particularly when performed through minimally invasive approaches.

The Bentall–De Bono operation remains the most versatile and predictable technique, offering consistently good surgical results. It should be considered the procedure of choice for managing complex aortic root pathology, especially for less experienced surgeons. Nevertheless, patients must be counseled regarding the need for lifelong anticoagulation when a mechanical prosthesis is used, or the risk of structural degeneration when a biological prosthesis is selected.

The Yacoub remodeling procedure reconstructs the sinuses of Valsalva using a prosthetic graft while preserving the native valve, resulting in more physiologic root dynamics due to the retention of native commissures and aortic wall support. However, to ensure long-term durability, additional annular stabilization is often required.

Modern cardiac surgery is moving toward minimally invasive and even ultraminimally invasive approaches. Techniques such as ministernotomy and mini-thoracotomy are gaining widespread acceptance, as they reduce surgical trauma, accelerate recovery, and enhance patient comfort without compromising outcomes – provided they are performed in experienced centers.

The success of minimally invasive aortic surgery strongly depends on the experience of the surgical team and the number of procedures performed. Careful preoperative imaging evaluation – including TTE and contrast-enhanced CTA – is essential for appropriate patient selection, ensuring optimal technique choice, and minimizing perioperative risk.

Properly selected patients can enjoy not only an excellent cosmetic outcome but also outstanding long-term clinical results. **Figure 20**.

Acknowledgments

The authors did not use generative AI for the article's creation; AI algorithms were used for the development of the chapter's outline and final editing only; the final content and scientific interpretation were fully reviewed and approved by the authors.

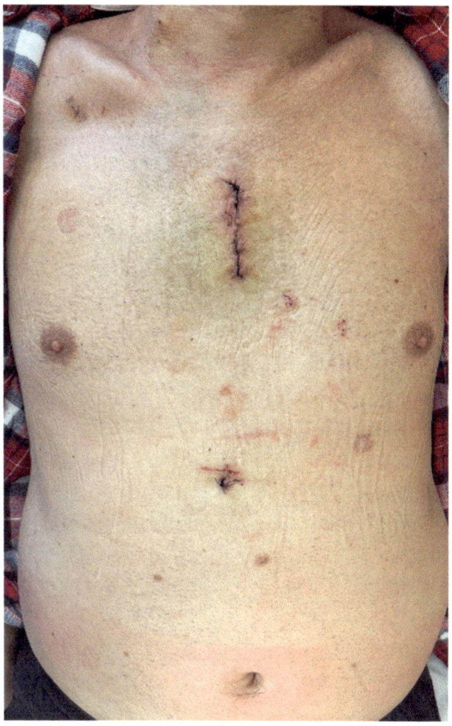

Figure 20.
Cosmetic effect after complex aortic root surgery.

Author details

Jakub Staromlynski[1,2*] and Piotr Suwalski[1,2]

1 Department of Cardiac Surgery and Transplantology, National Medical Institute of the Ministry of the Interior and Administration, Warsaw, Poland

2 Centre of Postgraduate Medical Education, Warsaw, Poland

*Address all correspondence to: jakubstaromlynski@gmail.com

References

[1] Salenger R, Lobdell K, Grant MC. Update on minimally invasive cardiac surgery and enhanced recovery after surgery. Current Opinion in Anaesthesiology. 2024;**37**(1):10–15. DOI: 10.1097/ACO.0000000000001322

[2] Guo MH, Fei LYN, Boodhwani M. Specialized thoracic aortic team is the next step in improving outcome in acute aortic dissection care. Journal of Thoracic Disease. 2020;**12**(10):6112–6114. DOI: 10.21037/jtd-2020-24

[3] Köpcke C, et al. Diagnostic value of chest radiography for thoracic aortic aneurysm. The European Radiology 2020;**30**:1670–1678

[4] Isselbacher EM, Preventza O, Hamilton Black III J, et al. ACC/AHA guideline for the diagnosis and management of aortic disease: A report of the American Heart Association/American College of Cardiology Joint Committee on Clinical Practice Guidelines. Circulation. 2022;**146**(24): e334–e482. DOI: 10.1161/CIR.0000000000001106

[5] Fogante M, Esposto Pirani P, Cela F, Alfonsi J, Tagliati C, Balardi L, Argalia G, Di Eusanio M, Schicchi N. Computed tomography imaging of thoracic aortic surgery: Distinguishing life-saving repairs from life-threatening complications. Journal of Imaging. 2025;**11**:119. DOI: 10.3390/jimaging11040119

[6] Staromłyński J, Kowalewski M, Sarnowski W, et al. Mini-David procedure. Procedural considerations. Kardiochir Torakochirurgia Pol. 2022;**19**(4):243–248. DOI: 10.5114/kitp.2022.122096

[7] CA Jr J, Siordia JA, Wood KL, Robinson DA, Knight PA. Right mini-thoracotomy Bentall procedure. Innovations: Technology and Techniques in Cardiothoracic and Vascular Surgery. 2018;**13**(5):328–331

[8] He X, Guo F, Li J, Li Y, Yan Y. The safety and feasibility of mini-invasive Bentall surgery via right anterior mini-thoracotomy. Journal of Thoracic Disease. 2024;**16**(5):2918–2926. DOI: 10.21037/jtd-23-1757

[9] Mazzolai L, Teixido-Tura G, Lanzi S, et al. ESC Guidelines for the management of peripheral arterial and aortic diseases. European Heart Journal. 2024;**45**(36):3538–3700. DOI: 10.1093/eurheartj/ehae179

[10] Paruchuri V, Salhab KF, Kuzmik GA, Gubernikoff G, Fang H, Rizzo JA, Elefteriades JA, et al. Aortic size distribution in the general population: Explaining the size paradox in aortic dissection. Cardiology. 2015;**131**(4):265–272. DOI: 10.1159/000381281

[11] Staromłyński J, Kowalówka A, Gocoł R, Hudziak D, Żurawska M, Nowak W, Pasierski M, Sarnowski W, Smoczyński R, Bartczak M, Brączkowski J, Sadecka S, Drobiński D, Deja M, Szymański P, Suwalski P, Kowalewski M. Comparative analysis of long-term outcomes in valve-sparing aortic root reimplantation: Full sternotomy versus mini-sternotomy approach. Journal of Clinical Medicine. 2024;**13**(9):2692. DOI: 10.3390/jcm13092692

[12] Paulenka Y, Lee C, Tawayha M, Dow S, Shah K, Henkin S, Mosleh W. From natural history to contemporary management of aortic diseases: A state-of-the-art review of thoracic aortic aneurysm. Cardiogenetics. 2023;**13**(4):154–172. DOI: 10.3390/cardiogenetics13040015

[13] Nguyen HC, Pham DT. Totally 3D endoscopic aortic valve replacement: Initial results and experience from a single center. Frontiers in Cardiovascular Medicine. 2024;**11**(1468452). DOI:10.3389/fcvm.2024.1468452

[14] Helms F, Deniz E, Krüger H, Zubarevich A, Schmitto JD, Poyanmehr R, Hinteregger M, Martens A, Weymann A, Ruhparwar A, et al. Minimally invasive approach for replacement of the ascending aorta towards the proximal aortic arch. Journal of Clinical Medicine. 2024;**13**(11):3274. DOI: 10.3390/jcm13113274

[15] Robinson E, Liu T, Whippo B, et al. Short-term outcomes in upper-hemi sternotomy for ascending and hemi-arch aortic repair with and without concomitant aortic valve replacement or repair. Asian Cardiovascular and Thoracic Annals. 2025;**33**:275–280

[16] Kirmani BH, Jones SG, Muir A, et al. Limited versus full sternotomy for aortic valve replacement. The Cochrane Database of Systematic Reviews. 2023;**12**(12):CD011793. DOI: 10.1002/14651858.CD011793.pub3

[17] Berretta P, Galeazzi M, Cefarelli M, *et al.* Minimally invasive approach: Is this the future of aortic surgery? Indian Journal of Thoracic and Cardiovascular Surgery. 2022;**38**(Suppl 1):171–182. DOI: 10.1007/s12055-021-01258-2

[18] Hamiko M, Salamate S, Nassari MA, Spaeth A, Sirat S, Doss M, Amer M, Silaschi M, Ahmad AE-S, Bakhtiary F. Totally endoscopic replacement of the ascending aorta and the aortic root including the aortic valve via right mini-thoracotomy: A multicenter study. Journal of Clinical Medicine. 2024;**13**:2648. DOI: 10.3390/jcm13092648

[19] Sicim H, Çaynak B. Open Seldinger technique in peripheral cannulation strategy for minimally invasive cardiac surgery. Journal Updates in Cardiovascular Medicine. 2024;**12**(4):133–141. DOI: 10.32596/jucvm.galenos.2024.2024-24-92

[20] Ma J, Wang H, Wang X, Hou X. Central (aortic) cannulation versus peripheral (axillary or femoral) cannulation in acute type a aortic dissections: A meta-analysis of comparative studies. Reviews in Cardiovascular Medicine. 2024;**25**(5):156. DOI: 10.31083/j.rcm2505156

[21] Yücel C, Kayalar N, Ketenciler S, Erentuğ V. Comparison of high aortic arch and other arterial cannulation types in ascending aortic pathologies. Journal of Surgery and Medicine. 2021;**5**(2):135–139. Available from: https://jsurgmed.com/article/view/757190

[22] David TE, Feindel CM. An aortic valve-sparing operation for patients with aortic incompetence and aneurysm of the ascending aorta. The Journal of Thoracic and Cardiovascular Surgery. 1992;**103**(4):617–622

[23] Schäfers HJ, Aicher D. Root remodeling for aortic root dilatation. Annals of Cardiothoracic Surgery. 2013;**2**(1):113–116. DOI: 10.3978/j.issn.2225-319X.2013.01.06

[24] Schäfers HJ, Schmied W, Marom G, Aicher D. Cusp height in aortic valves. The Journal of Thoracic and Cardiovascular Surgery. 2013;**146**: 269–274

[25] Shraer N, Youssefi P, Zacek P, et al. Bicuspid valve repair outcomes are improved with reduction and stabilization of sinotubular junction and annulus with external annuloplasty. Journal of Thoracic and Cardiovascular Surgery. 2024;**168**(1):60–73.e6. DOI: 10.1016/j.jtcvs.2022.11.021

[26] Federspiel JM, Ehrlich T, Abeln K, Schäfers HJ. Aortic annuloplasty: Subcommissural, intra-annular suture techniques, external and internal rings. JTCVS Techniques. 2021;7:98–102. DOI: 10.1016/j.xjtc.2020.12.044

[27] Woo YJ. New horizons in aortic valve repair. JTCVS Techniques. 2021;7:71. DOI: 10.1016/j.xjtc.2021.04.018

[28] De Paulis R, Torre M, Scaffa R. Straight tube versus Valsalva graft for valve-sparing operation. Annals of Cardiothoracic Surgery. 2023;**12**(4):358–360. DOI: 10.21037/acs-2023-avs2-10

[29] Svensson LG. The art of aortic valve repair. JTCVS Techniques. 2021;7:121–125. DOI: 10.1016/j.xjtc.2021.01.030

[30] David TE, David CM, Feindel CM, Manlhiot C. Reimplantation of the aortic valve at 20 years. The Journal of Thoracic and Cardiovascular Surgery. 2017;**153**(2):232–238. DOI: 10.1016/j.jtcvs.2016.10.081

[31] Westaby S, Katsumata T, Vaccari G. Aortic root replacement with coronary button re-implantation: Low risk and predictable outcome. European Journal of Cardio-Thoracic Surgery. 2000;**17**(3):259–265. DOI: 10.1016/S1010-7940(00)00347-X

[32] Urbanski PP, Heinz N, Zhan X, Hijazi H, Zacher M, Diegeler A. Modified bio-Bentall procedure: 10-year experience. European Journal of Cardio-Thoracic Surgery. 2010;**37**(6):1317–1321. DOI: 10.1016/j.ejcts.2009.12.017

[33] Botea R, Lavie-Badie Y, Goicea A, Porterie J, Marcheix B. Early and midterm outcomes of a bentall operation using an all-biological valved BioConduit™. Journal of Cardiothoracic Surgery. 2022;**17**(1):325. DOI: 10.1186/s13019-022-02073-5

[34] Song L, et al. Bentall procedure in the small aortic root after prior aortic valve operations. The Annals of Thoracic Surgery 2020;**110**:e241–e243

[35] Galeone A, Gardellini J, Perrone F, Di Nicola V, Dian G, Di Gaetano R, Luciani GB. Mechanical versus biological bentall procedure: A propensity-score matching analysis of 548 consecutive patients. Journal of Clinical Medicine. 2025;**14**(14):5105. DOI: 10.3390/jcm14145105

[36] Sá MP, Tasoudis P, Jacquemyn X, et al. Long-term outcomes of patients undergoing aortic root replacement with mechanical versus bioprosthetic valves: Meta-analysis of reconstructed time-to-event data. Journal of the American Heart Association. 2023;**12**(18):e030629. DOI: 10.1161/JAHA.123.030629

[37] CY C, CY C, Chang FC, et al. Mechanical versus bioprosthetic aortic valve replacement in patients undergoing bentall procedure. Journal of the American Heart Association.

2024;**13**(1):e030328. DOI: 10.1161/JAHA.123.030328

[38] Calderon-Rojas R, Bagameri G, Schaff HV, et al. Early experience with a prefabricated bioprosthetic aortic valved conduit: The first 100. JTCVS Open. 2025;**26**:34–43

[39] Bartus K, Bavaria JE, Thourani VH, Xu K, Keuffel EL. Structural hemodynamic valve deterioration durability of RESILIA-tissue versus contemporary aortic bioprostheses. Journal of Comparative Effectiveness Research. 2023;**12**(3):e220180. DOI: 10.2217/cer-2022-0180

[40] Yan TD. Mini-bentall procedure: The "French Cuff" technique. The Annals of Thoracic Surgery. 2016;**101**(2):780–782. DOI: 10.1016/j.athoracsur.2015.06.092

[41] Wilson-Smith AR, Wilson-Smith CJ, Strode Smith J, et al. The outcomes of three decades of the David and Yacoub procedures in bicuspid aortic valve patients-a systematic review and meta-analysis. Annals of Cardiothoracic Surgery. 2023;**12**(4):286–294. DOI: 10.21037/acs-2023-avs2-19

[42] Schäfers HJ. Aortic root remodeling: A valid option. The Journal of Thoracic and Cardiovascular Surgery. 2025;**169**(4):1210–1213.e1. DOI: 10.1016/j.jtcvs.2024.05.012

[43] Sromicki J, Van Hemelrijck M, Schmiady MO, Greutmann M, Bonassin Tempesta F, Mestres CA, Vogt PR, Carrel TP, Holubec T. Twenty-five year experience with aortic valve-sparing root replacement in a single teaching center. Frontiers in Cardiovascular Medicine. 2023;**10**:1104149. DOI: 10.3389/fcvm.2023.1104149

[44] Guenther TM, Godoy L, Chen SA, Rodriguez VM. Homograft aortic root replacement with modified Cabrol extension using cryopreserved femoral artery for bioprosthetic aortic valve endocarditis. JTCVS Techniques. 2020;**4**:65–67. DOI: 10.1016/j.xjtc.2020.08.019

[45] Williams ML, Brookes JDL, Jaya JS, Tan E. Homograft versus valves and valved conduits for extensive aortic valve endocarditis with aortic root involvement/destruction: A systematic review and meta-analysis. Aorta (Stamford). 2022;**10**(2):43–51. DOI: 10.1055/s-0042-1743110

Chapter 4

Perspective Chapter: Sliding Rail Technique (Mandelli's), A Better Method to Repair Thoracoabdominal Aortic Aneurysms with Controlled Release Fenestrated Endoprosthesis

Nilo César Barbosa Mandelli and Felipe Figueiró Teixeira

Abstract

Thoracoabdominal aortic aneurysm (TAAA) remains one of the most complex and high-risk pathologies in vascular surgery, often involving the visceral and renal branches and demanding precise technical solutions. The continuous evolution of endovascular repair has transformed TAAA management, progressing from early infrarenal Endovascular aneurysm repair (EVAR) and thoracic endovascular aortic repair (TEVAR) to advanced fenestrated and branched endografts. However, despite significant innovation, conventional fenestrated endovascular aortic repair (FEVAR) and branched endovascular aortic repair (BEVAR) procedures continue to face challenges such as difficult visceral vessel catheterization, prolonged operative times, and high radiation and contrast exposure. The sliding rail technique (Mandelli) represents a novel and refined approach designed to overcome these limitations. By repositioning the working zone outside the aneurysmal segment, utilizing strategic "sliding rails" with guidewires and sheaths, and employing controlled-release endografts, this technique enhances precision, stability, and procedural efficiency. It simplifies visceral catheterization even in hostile anatomies, reduces fluoroscopy and contrast use, and improves reproducibility among surgical teams. This chapter provides a comprehensive narrative on the historical evolution of complex aortic repair, the rationale behind the sliding rail technique, and detailed technical steps for its implementation. It also discusses the theoretical advantages, clinical implications, and future perspectives for integrating this method with next-generation endovascular technologies. The sliding rail technique emerges as an important contribution to the field, offering a safer, more predictable, and potentially more durable endovascular solution for complex thoracoabdominal aneurysm repair.

Keywords: fenestrated endovascular aortic aneurysm repair (FEVAR), thoracoabdominal aortic aneurysms (TAAAs), juxtarenal aneurysms, double brachial access, controlled-release fenestrated endoprosthesis

1. Introduction

1.1 The TAAA: A central challenge in modern vascular surgery

Thoracoabdominal aneurysm (TAAA) represents one of the most challenging pathologies in vascular surgery, characterized by involvement of the descending thoracic aorta and abdominal aorta, including the emergence of visceral and renal branches. Its anatomical complexity and extent make treatment a matter of high morbidity and mortality rates. The Crawford Classification, with its Types I–IV (1986), and the Safi/Miller modification, which introduced Type V (1999) [1, 2], serve as the fundamental anatomical basis for risk stratification and treatment planning. This understanding is crucial to guide decision-making, given the high probability of serious complications such as spinal cord ischemia, renal failure, and other adverse perioperative events.

1.2 The continuous evolution of endovascular treatment: From classical EVAR to fenestrated and branched solutions

The field of aortic surgery has witnessed a remarkable revolution with the rise of endovascular treatment. The starting point of this journey was the endovascular repair of infrarenal aneurysms (EVAR), introduced by Parodi in 1991, followed by the endovascular repair of descending thoracic aortic aneurysms (TEVAR) by Dake in 1994. These procedures transformed the management of aneurysms, offering less invasive alternatives to open surgery.

The need to treat more complex aneurysms, involving the emergence of visceral and renal branches, drove the development of more sophisticated endoprostheses. Fenestrated endoprostheses (FEVAR) emerged, designed to preserve perfusion of these target vessels through custom openings in the prosthesis body. Devices such as the Cook Zenith® Fenestrated (ZFEN) represented a significant advance in this regard, obtaining FDA approval in 2012. Subsequently, branched endoprostheses (BEVAR) and, more recently, multibranched off-the-shelf (OTS) devices, such as the t-Branch, gained traction, with multicenter series published between 2013 and 2022. In a notable breakthrough, the GORE EXCLUDER ALTO, in addition, obtained FDA approval in 2024, further expanding the therapeutic arsenal for complex TAAA.

Despite these remarkable advances, conventional FEVAR/BEVAR techniques still face considerable challenges. The complexity and time-consuming nature of visceral vessel catheterization, especially in unfavorable anatomies or those with steep angulations, can lead to prolonged radiation exposure and increased contrast use, in addition to a potentially high reintervention rate.

1.3 Sliding rail technique (mandelli): A new approach for complex TAAAs

Given these obstacles, the Sliding Rail Technique (Mandelli) emerges as a promising innovation, designed to overcome the limitations of conventional FEVAR/BEVAR approaches. This technique aims to optimize stent positioning and manipulation, especially in complex aortic anatomies, striving for greater operational simplicity, predictability, and safety in the implantation of fenestrated controlled-release stents.

2. Historical basis and evolution of complex aortic repair

2.1 Early open aortic surgery

The history of aortic aneurysm treatment dates back to the 1950s, when the term "thoracoabdominal aneurysm" was described by Charles Rob at the Royal Society of Surgery, followed by the first reports of treatment by DeBakey and Cooley. For many decades, open surgery was the "gold standard" for repairing these aneurysms, a major procedure that required spinal cord and renal protection, such as cerebrospinal fluid (CSF) drainage and the use of moderate hypothermia to mitigate the inherent risks. The complexity of TAAA was so great that the famous book "Rutherford, the Bible of aortic surgery," devoted only four pages to the topic.

2.2 The endovascular revolution and the expansion of indications

The true revolution in the management of aortic aneurysms began with the introduction of endovascular techniques. Infrarenal EVAR, described by Parodi in 1991, and TEVAR for the descending thoracic aorta, described by Dake in 1994, broke new ground, offering less invasive alternatives to open surgery [3, 4]. However, the application of these techniques to complex aneurysms involving visceral and renal vessels required the development of more advanced technologies.

This demand, as well as advancements, led to the emergence of fenestrated and branched stent grafts. Important milestones include the first fenestrated adrenal covered stent, described by Browne et al. in 1999, which allowed the preservation of a renal artery. Shortly thereafter, Anderson et al. (2001) developed the multifenestrated graft capable of incorporating both renal arteries and the superior mesenteric artery (SMA) [5, 6]. In the same year, Chuter et al. presented the first multibranched device for type III TAAA, marking the beginning of the branched stent graft era [7]. Between 2008 and 2011, there was standardization and early-phase studies for BEVAR/branched devices. The FDA approval of the Cook Zenith Fenestrated (ZFEN) in 2012 and the subsequent consolidation of multibranched OTS devices, such as the t-Branch (2013–2022), significantly expanded treatment options [8, 9]. More recently, the approval of the GORE EXCLUDER TAMBE in 2024 further solidified the position of endovascular repair for TAAA by offering a multibranched OTS device [10].

2.3 Persistent challenges and the quest for optimization

Despite technological advances, endovascular repair of TAAA still presents challenges. Catheterization of visceral vessels remains one of the most critical and technically demanding aspects, especially in complex anatomies with pronounced aortic neck angulations. The need for multiple cannulations can significantly prolong procedure time, increase radiation exposure for the patient and team, and require a larger volume of contrast, increasing the risk of complications.

Complications such as limb ischemia, renal dysfunction, and reperfusion injury are valid concerns, often associated with prolonged procedures. Furthermore, the literature suggests that reintervention rates in FEVAR/BEVAR may be higher in the long term, justifying the search for more reproducible and safe methods. These obstacles justify the continued innovation and development of techniques such as the sliding rail technique.

3. Technical choice of endoprosthesis type for TAAA treatment

3.1 Justification for the use of fenestrated versus branched endoprosthesis

In narrow paravisceral aortas (<30 mm), fenestrated stents are preferred because devices with branches (side cuffs + bridging stents) "invade" the lumen and compete for space, increasing the risk of crowding, stent kinking/compression, and loss of patency in small aortas. Fenestrated devices, on the other hand, align tangentially to the ostia and use lower-profile stents, preserving the effective ductus diameter and facilitating sealing. Furthermore, instructions for use and clinical series indicate that branched devices require a minimum visceral segment diameter of approximately ≥25 mm (e.g., T-Branch) and recommend avoiding external branches when the lumen is <25 mm, especially if there is calcification or a long, narrow segment – a situation in which the fenestrated strategy tends to be safer. Additionally, it is important that, in fenestrations, balloon-expanded stents for renal/mesenteric arteries have typical diameters of ~5–6.5 mm, contributing to less intraluminal protrusion in small aortas.

3.2 Oversize planning

In aortic necks <30 mm, oversizing (20%) for proximal sealing (e.g., 30→36 mm) is common practice. However, when the lumen needs to be reduced to ~20 mm to accommodate a branched EVAR (BEVAR), wall shear stress (WSS) increases sharply (WSS $1/D^3$) and Reynolds number (Re) increases (Re 1/D), favoring shear layers at the neck and poststenotic turbulence as diameter loss approaches/exceeds ~50% (making ≥70% stenosis more likely). Furthermore, patient-specific simulations show that BEVAR markedly increases aortic time-averaged WSS (TAWSS) (≈ +200%) compared to FEVAR (fenestrated), reinforcing that, in small aortas, solutions that preserve the effective ductus diameter tend to disrupt flow less. Finally, instructions for use (IFU) of stent grafts with branches define proximal necks as 24–30 mm (e.g., t-Branch 34 mm for 24–30 mm) and, in the case of inner branches (E-nside), recommend 27–30 mm for the proximal 33 mm segment – criteria that restrict the use of branches in necks <30 mm and, in this scenario, favor fenestrations [11, 12].

4. Rationale and fundamental principles of the sliding rail technique

The sliding rail technique (Mandelli) was developed as a direct response to persistent challenges in endovascular repair of complex TAAA, aiming to improve procedural predictability and safety [13]. Its innovation is based on three fundamental premises:

4.1 The three innovative premises of technique

- **Repositioning outside the hostile zone:** Unlike conventional approaches, which often require manipulation and catheterization of the visceral branches in an already complex and hostile aortic zone (such as the aneurysm area), the sliding rail technique advocates the initial positioning of the stent graft in a straight, healthy segment of the aorta, either thoracic or abdominal, outside the origin of the visceral branches. This strategic positioning optimizes working angles and provides more precise control of the stent graft before its final deployment, facilitating subsequent steps and reducing tissue tension.

- **Sliding rails:** This technique employs the strategic placement of sheaths and rigid guidewires in the renal and visceral branches, typically from brachial access points. Once anchored, these wires and sheaths serve as "sliding rails," guiding the stent graft in a controlled and predictable manner to its ideal position. This controlled caudal traction mechanism allows the stent graft to "slide" smoothly over the guidewires, minimizing the risk of misalignment or unwanted rotation.

- **Use of controlled-release endoprostheses:** The effectiveness of the sliding rail technique is amplified by the use of recapturable and repositionable fenestrated endoprostheses. These devices allow for fine adjustments to the prosthesis' position before final release, which is crucial for ensuring precise alignment of the fenestrations with the visceral vessel ostia. The repositioning capability significantly reduces technical failures and fluoroscopy time, contributing to a safer and more efficient procedure.

4.2 Theoretical advantages and potential benefits

The combination of these premises gives the Sliding Rail Technique a series of significant clinical advantages:

- **Greater operational simplicity and predictability:** By shifting the initial manipulation of the stent graft to a less critical area, the technique simplifies the visceral catheterization process, which is traditionally one of the most challenging aspects of FEVAR/BEVAR. This results in a smoother learning curve for surgeons and increases the reproducibility of the technique in a variety of complex anatomical scenarios.

- **Reduced exposure and procedure time:** Optimizing surgical steps and increasing the predictability of stent placement significantly reduce operative time and fluoroscopy time. Consequently, there is reduced radiation exposure for both the patient and the surgical team, as well as a reduction in the volume of iodinated contrast agent used, which is particularly beneficial for patients with compromised renal function [14, 15].

- **Less aggressive access:** The technique is adaptable to the use of ultrasound-guided punctures and the selection of appropriate calibers for vascular access, which can reduce the incidence of local complications such as hematomas and pseudoaneurysms. Brachial access, although complex, is a common route for complex aortic interventions.

- **Synergy with new technologies:** The sliding rail technique aligns perfectly with the evolution of repositionable and controlled-release endovascular devices, enhancing their benefits and establishing a new paradigm in the clinical practice of endovascular repair of TAAA.

5. Technical details of the sliding rail technique

Successful application of the sliding rail technique requires meticulous planning and precise technical execution.

5.1 Image-based preoperative planning

Planning is the cornerstone of any complex endovascular repair. Multislice computed tomography angiogram (CT angiogram) with 3D reconstruction is the diagnostic tool of choice and is indispensable for the preoperative evaluation of TAAA. This method, considered worldwide to be the best for prestent graft placement evaluation, provides essential measurements for selecting and sizing the ideal prosthesis for each patient.

DICOM image postprocessing technology enables vessel centerline reconstruction, stretched visualization, and accurate measurements of aorta and target vessel diameters and lengths. This includes determining the diameters and angles of target vessels (renal arteries, superior mesenteric artery, celiac trunk [CT]), which is essential for selecting endoprostheses and bridging stents (fenestrated or branched). OsiriX, an open-source program for Mac OS X, additionally offers most of the tools available on powerful workstations, including the ability to perform multiplanar reconstructions and centerline calculation, allowing for more reliable measurements, especially when manually corrected for deviations from automated algorithms.

Planning, in addition, includes determining the best arterial access points (femoral and brachial), considering the anatomy and tortuosity of the vessels to ensure safe navigation of catheters and introducers. Proper planning can reduce surgical time and radiation exposure.

5.2 Vascular accesses

Vascular accesses are crucial for performing the technique:

- **Femoral access:** Generally used to introduce the main endoprosthesis into the aorta. It can be done via dissection or percutaneously (using a sealing device).

- **Bilateral brachial access:** Used for catheterization and implantation of bridging stents in the visceral branches. The recommendation is to perform a bilateral cubital fossa puncture in the case of two fenestrae. In specific cases, a double puncture is performed in the brachial artery: the first over the distal humerus and the second 10 cm above (**Figure 1**), with ultrasound-guided or

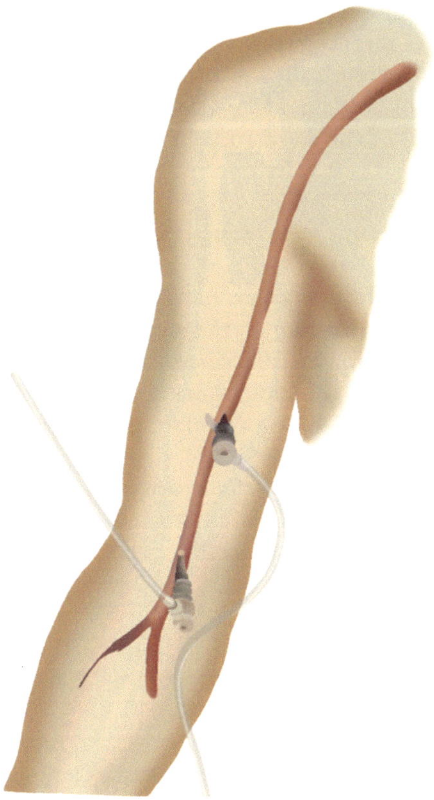

Figure 1.
Artistic rendering of the double puncture in the right brachial artery. The first puncture is placed at the level of the medial epicondyle of the humerus, followed by a second puncture approximately 10 cm above the first.

fluoroscopy-guided puncture, using the inferior puncture guide as a reference. Careful handling is necessary to prevent local complications, such as hematoma and pseudoaneurysm.

- **Axillary access:** Access via dissection is always recommended. It is used as an alternative to double brachial access or for greater support in cases of type II or III aortic arch. We chose to use a 12 F/45 cm sheath because the passage of multiple sheaths increases the risk of atheroembolism and, therefore, is less harmful.

5.3 Sequential steps of the sliding rail technique

The sequence of steps in the technique is designed to optimize the positioning of the endoprosthesis:

5.3.1 Initial positioning of the endoprosthesis

The procedure begins with the placement of a Lunderquist-type guidewire in the aortic arch. The endoprosthesis is then advanced and temporarily positioned in a healthy area of the aorta, proximal to the fenestrations, typically at the level of vertebrae T8 to T9. This initial positioning creates an optimized working space for the catheterization of the target vessels.

As we frequently use a stent called Apolo® (nano endoluminal) that has release control, retraction control, and dual free-flow, this facilitates anterograde entry into the proximal portion of the stent (brachial route). We then begin the release process until the first fenestra is fully open.

5.3.2 Creation of greater support for catheterization of target vessels

Then, the brachial introducers are exchanged for long sheaths — 6 F/90 cm, 7 F/90 cm, or 8 F/90 cm (depending on the stent-bridge profile) — up to the T8 level. In cases where we opt for axillary dissection, these long sheaths are passed through the 12 F/45 cm sheath. We do not use the 9 F/90 cm sheath because it is not possible to pass it along the 0.035/260 Amplatz guide through the 12 F sheath.

5.3.3 Catheterization of the CT and superior mesenteric

A 5 F/125 cm catheter is used because, as we use 90 cm sheaths, 100 cm catheters make catheterization difficult.

After catheterization of the fenestra, the arch is positioned for oblique viewing. The CT scan has already assessed its position in relation to the vertebral body and determined the best angle for visualization, whether it is oblique left or right, and at what angle. No contrast has been used to date.

A breath-hold is performed with 10 ml of contrast. Any of the arteries can be visualized. In this case, we will report a 4-fenestrated endoprosthesis, the first being the CT. The next step, after catheterizing the artery, is to place an Amplatz guide, preferably with a 1 cm tip, leaving it in the splenic artery to prevent further injury from the guide. We start on the right side of the upper limb (UL). We secure the guide in this artery, removing the long sheath from this guide. We now pass either through another puncture in the UL or through the 12 F sheath, leaving it alone. It will be used to lower the sheath after treating the right renal artery.

Remember that in the UL, two long sheaths should never be used simultaneously on the same side. When starting the puncture on the side that will be the CT, through the proximal puncture, after passing the guide through the trunk, the long sheath is removed, and a short 10 cm sheath is inserted. Because they are not wired, when passing the lower sheath, they collapse, and there is no bleeding around the proximal puncture. On the same side, when passing the long sheath, it now enters through the distal puncture, and this remains in the artery to form the rail for the endoprosthesis's descent (sliding rail).

Now, in the UL, descend in the same way as on the right, opening the stent further. Remember that our stent can be opened and closed to help catheterize the superior mesenteric (SM) fenestra. Perform another angiography with another 10 ml of contrast. Catheterize the SM, and, like the CT, leave the guide alone.

5.3.4 Catheterization of the renal branches

Through the brachial access, after catheterization of the renal fenestrae, rigid Amplatz guide wires with a 1 cm tip are advanced. The sheath introducer is placed to prevent a step when passing through the prosthesis fenestra. After passing the sheath, the arch is positioned, and with 10 ml of contrast, the renal artery is visualized.

Once the renal artery is catheterized, the Amplatz guidewire is inserted (**Figure 2A**, **B**). Remember that in renal arteries, it is mandatory to use a guidewire with the rigid part starting 1 cm from the tip, as renal arteries are on average three to four cm long, and using larger guidewires will lose support and cause damage to the distal artery. The catheter is removed, and the sheath tip is inserted to guide it two to three cm into the renal artery (**Figure 2C**). The sheath introducer is removed, leaving the sheath with the Amplatz guidewire inside.

The procedure is then repeated on the contralateral renal artery. It is crucial to ensure that the sheaths do not cross (the right access sheath on the right renal artery and the left access sheath on the left renal artery) to prevent trapping the stent's nitinol mesh.

5.3.5 Controlled caudal traction and rotation of the endoprosthesis

With the Amplatz guidewires and sheaths in the renal arteries acting as a "sliding rail," the Apolo® stent graft is pulled caudally and carefully rotated to its correct final position (**Figure 2D, Figure 3, Figure 4**). This movement aligns the fenestrations of the graft with the ostia of the target vessels, avoiding the risk of the geometry of the fenestrae and branches becoming misaligned, causing

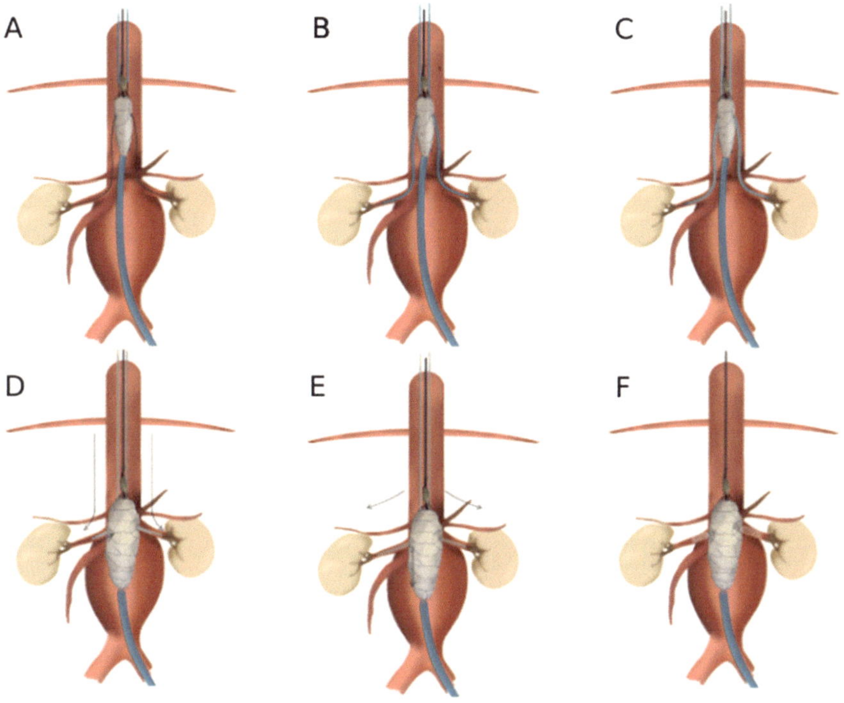

Figure 2.
Artistic rendering of the complete procedure. After positioning the endograft in the healthy aorta to optimize the working space for catheterization of the target vessels. A- The renal arteries were catheterized with a stiff guidewire. B- the 5F Vert catheter was advanced to the renal arteries with the goal of replacing the stiff guidewire with a super-stiff guidewire. C- Proximal advancement of the introducer sheaths under the guidance of an Amplatz wire. Confirmation of the proper positioning of the sheaths in the renal arteries, without crossing them and without entangling the nitinol mesh. D- Distal traction of the system was performed with rotation and sliding of the endograft along the sheath tracks until proper positioning was achieved. E- Release of the diameter restrainers. F- Implantation of the bridging stents.

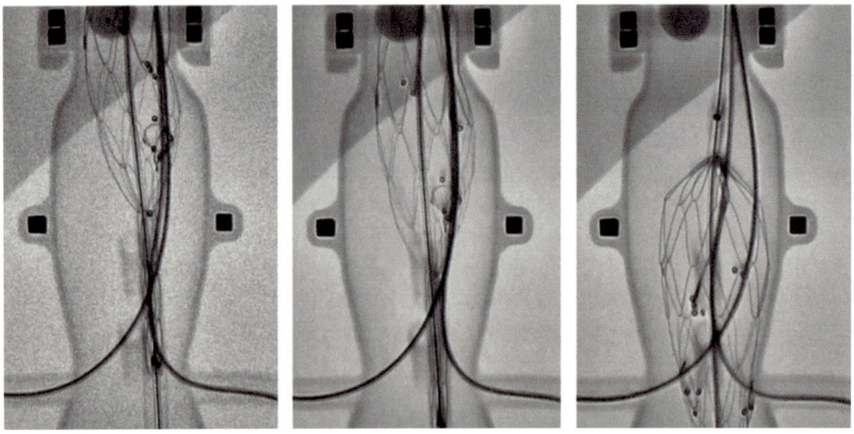

Figure 3.
In vitro representation of the Mandelli Sliding Rail Technique. The sequence of images allows us to observe the rotation of the endoprosthesis during sliding into the appropriate position.

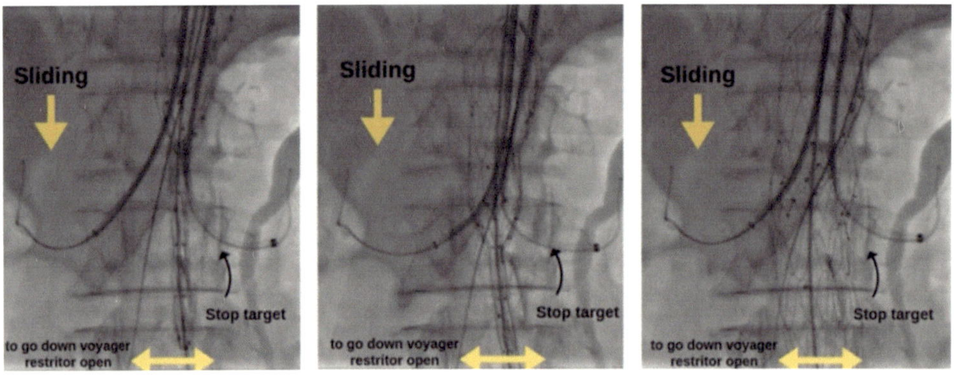

Figure 4.
Radiographic representation of the Mandelli Sliding Rail Technique. The image on the right shows us, after performing the maneuver, the release of the endoprosthesis diameter 60% restrictor.

angulation that could subsequently fracture or occlude the stent-bridge. In vitro and radiographic representations clearly demonstrate this rotation and seating.

5.3.6 Releasing the diameter restrictors

Once the stent graft is in the ideal position and aligned, the diameter restrictors are released (**Figure 2E**), allowing the graft to fully expand as well as seal proximally. It's important to note that, at this point, the stent graft is restricted to 40% of its diameter. The Apolo® stent graft, as mentioned above, has a restrictor® and the Voyager® system.

5.3.7 Implantation of bridge stents

The bridging stents are implanted first in the renal arteries (due to the prior positioning of the sheaths) and then in the superior mesenteric artery and CT, as planned (**Figure 2F**).

It's important to note that after the stent is released, the balloon is withdrawn and further inflated (a flaring maneuver) to increase the proximal diameter, helping to prevent future disconnection. The sheath is then lowered over the deflated balloon to prevent it from bumping into the stent and pushing it inward, disconnecting it from the fenestra. A follow-up angiogram is then performed, and the sheath is removed.

The removed sheaths will be slowly replaced on the Amplatz wires, located in the CT and SM, passing through the fenestrae; then, the same stent placement sequence is performed, with control angiography and stent flare.

5.3.8 Implantation of bridge stents

After this, the entire stent graft is released, first by removing the Voyager® system, followed by releasing the free-flow system. The stent graft, at this stage, establishes a neoneck below the renal arteries for implantation of the bifurcated stent graft. In highly angled necks, we plan the longest length of the fenestrated body to prevent the junction with the bifurcated body from being in the curve. This process is performed to ensure contact between at least three contact stents from both stent grafts, totaling four to six cm of neck.

5.3.9 Final control angiography

A control angiogram is performed to confirm the absence of dissections, endoleaks, and the patency of all visceral vessels before the removal of catheters and sheaths (**Figure** 5).

5.4 Essential technical care

During the entire procedure, some technical precautions are crucial:

- Ensuring that the hems do not cross is essential to prevent complications.

- Confirm free movement of the wires in relation to the nitinol mesh of the endoprosthesis to prevent entrapment.

- Maintain constant monitoring of access sites to detect and prevent possible complications, such as hematomas or pseudoaneurysms.

6. Advantages and clinical benefits of the sliding rail technique

The sliding rail technique offers a series of advantages and clinical benefits that position it as a significant advancement in the treatment of complex TAAAs.

6.1 Optimization of visceral catheterization and increased reproducibility

The sliding rail technique's greatest advantage lies in its operational simplicity, which facilitates catheterization of visceral vessels, even in complex and angled anatomies – one of the greatest challenges of conventional FEVAR/BEVAR techniques. This simplicity translates into greater predictability and reproducibility,

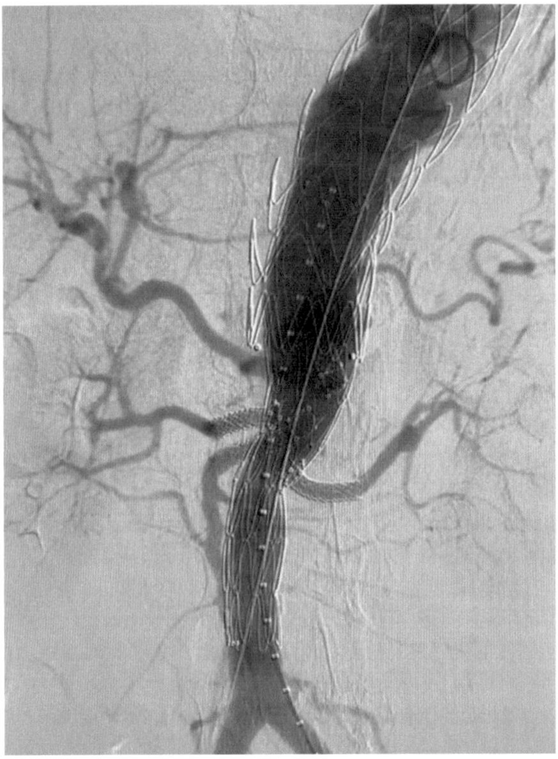

Figure 5.
Postoperative Aortography of the complete procedure. Implant the fenestrated visceral component inside the thoracic endoprosthesis implanted previously for the treatment of a thoracic aneurysm by sliding rail technique.

allowing the technique to be successfully applied in a wider range of anatomical TAAA scenarios, including Crawford types I–IV.

6.2 Reduction of time and exposure

Process optimization and predictability of endoprosthesis positioning lead to a significant reduction in operative time and fluoroscopy time. Consequently, there is less radiation exposure for both the patient and the surgical team. Furthermore, the volume of iodinated contrast agent used is reduced, which is a substantial benefit, especially for patients with preexisting renal impairment or those who will undergo multiple procedures over the course of their lives.

6.3 Impact on perioperative morbidity

- **Spinal cord ischemia:** Spinal cord protection is a primary concern in extensive aortic repairs. Although physiological strategies such as CSF drainage, maintenance of permissive hypertension, and segmental aortic perfusion (TASP) are crucial, the sliding rail technique may indirectly contribute to reducing spinal cord ischemia by decreasing aortic occlusion time and segmental vessel manipulation. Staging endovascular repair may, in addition, limit the incidence of spinal cord ischemia.

- **Renal insufficiency:** Minimizing visceral ischemia time and contrast volume are protective factors against acute kidney injury, a common complication in complex aortic repairs.

- **Access complications:** Emphasis on less invasive, ultrasound-guided access techniques, such as brachial punctures, may lead to a lower incidence of local complications at the puncture sites.

6.4 Durability and medium-term results

Although long-term studies are still ongoing, the logic behind the sliding rail technique suggests that the precision in positioning and stability of the fenestrations, ensured by the "sliding rail" methodology and the use of controlled-release endoprostheses, may contribute to the durability of the repair.

This is expected to result in low rates of stenosis, occlusion, or disconnection of visceral branches. The ability to address most complications with minimally invasive secondary interventions is, in addition, an advantage, facilitating long-term management.

7. Limitations and challenges

Despite the promising advantages of the sliding rail technique, it is essential to recognize its limitations and the challenges inherent in its application, ensuring a balanced perspective on its role in aortic surgery.

7.1 Learning curve and necessary experience

Although the technique is designed to offer greater operational simplicity and reproducibility, it requires considerable familiarity and experience on the part of the surgeon. The coordinated manipulation of brachial accesses (which may be double) and multiple sheaths and guidewires requires dexterity and a thorough understanding of vascular anatomy. Expertise in interpreting complex 3D images and using controlled-release devices is equally essential. For these reasons, the sliding rail technique should preferably be implemented and practiced in high-volume centers by experienced surgical teams capable of handling the inherent complexity of TAAA and the nuances of the technique.

7.2 Dependency on specific devices

The full effectiveness of the sliding rail technique is intrinsically linked to the availability and access to controlled-release, repositionable, fenestrated stents. The technology behind these devices is crucial to enabling the fine adjustments and positioning precision that characterize the technique. In some regions or institutions, the availability of these cutting-edge devices may be limited, thereby restricting the applicability of the technique.

7.3 Possible specific complications

Although the sliding rail technique aims to reduce complications associated with conventional techniques, the intrinsic complexity of TAAAs means that risks such as spinal cord ischemia, visceral vessel injury, or access site complications can still occur. Managing these events requires close monitoring and an experienced team. The literature, in addition, documents potential complications associated with UL access for complex aortic interventions, which, although minimized by the technique, require attention.

8. Future perspectives and integration in the aortic surgery scenario

The future of the sliding rail technique is promising, and its continued integration into the aortic surgery landscape will depend on research, validation, and adaptation.

8.1 Need for robust multicenter evaluations

To establish the Sliding Rail Technique as a therapeutic standard, robust multicenter studies are essential. These evaluations should compare the technique with conventional FEVAR/BEVAR, analyzing long-term clinical outcomes, procedure time, radiation exposure, morbidity, and mortality on a larger scale. Obtaining high-level evidence is crucial to guide clinical practice and widespread adoption [16, 17].

8.2 Integration with recapturable OTS devices

The sliding rail technique has great potential for combination with the next generation of recapturable OTS stent grafts. The synergy between the technique's predictable positioning and the flexibility of these devices could make TAAA treatment even more accessible, standardized, and rapid, expanding the range of patients eligible for endovascular treatment.

8.3 Expansion to challenging scenarios

Investigating the application of the sliding rail technique in emergency situations, such as ruptured aneurysms or anatomies considered extreme, is a crucial area of research. In these scenarios, the technique's simplicity and predictability may become even more valuable, offering a potentially faster and safer therapeutic option in high-risk settings.

8.4 Research focused on spinal cord protection

It is essential that future studies analyze the specific impact of the sliding rail technique on preventing spinal cord ischemia. This investigation should be conducted in conjunction with other neuroprotective strategies, such as segmental aortic perfusion (TASP) and CSF drainage, to fully understand how the technique contributes to neurological safety in extensive TAAA repairs.

8.5 Impact on education and training

The sliding rail technique's potential for simplification could positively influence training paradigms in endovascular surgery. By making TAAA repair more accessible, the technique can empower a greater number of vascular surgeons, always with due emphasis on specialized training and understanding of the learning curve required for mastery.

9. Conclusion

The sliding rail technique (Mandelli) represents a significant milestone in the evolution of endovascular surgery for TAAAs. By optimizing visceral catheterization, reducing procedure time, and increasing reproducibility, this innovation emerges as a crucial step in establishing endovascular repair as a robust and preferred therapeutic standard for complex TAAA.

This is a promising approach that, with continued validation through multicenter studies and the integration of new technologies, has the potential to redefine the way we treat complex aortic aneurysms, especially in referral centers. We are committed to continuing to improve and disseminate this technique to provide the best possible care for our patients.

Author details

Nilo César Barbosa Mandelli* and Felipe Figueiró Teixeira
Vascular and Endovascular Surgery, IC-FUC: Instituto de Cardiologia, Porto Alegre, Brazil

*Address all correspondence to: mdncbm@gmail.com

References

[1] Crawford ES, Crawford JL, Safi HJ, Coselli JS, Hess KR, Brooks B, et al. Thoracoabdominal aortic aneurysms: Preoperative and intraoperative factors determining results in 605 patients. Journal of Vascular Surgery. 1986;**3** (3):389–404. DOI: 10.1067/mva.1986.avs0030389

[2] Safi HJ, Miller CC. Spinal cord protection in descending thoracic and thoracoabdominal aortic repair. The Annals of Thoracic Surgery. 1999;**67** (6):1937–1942. DOI: 10.1016/s0003-4975(99)00397-5

[3] Parodi JC, Barone HD. Transfemoral intraluminal graft implantation for abdominal aortic aneurysms. Annals of Vascular Surgery. 1991;**5**(6):491–499. DOI: 10.1007/BF02015271

[4] Dake MD, Miller DC, Semba CP, Mitchell RS, Walker PJ, Liddell RP, et al. Transluminal placement of endovascular stent-grafts for the treatment of descending thoracic aortic aneurysms. New England Journal of Medicine. 1994;**331**(26):1729–1734. DOI: 10.1056/NEJM199412293312601

[5] Faruqi RM, Chuter TA, Reilly LM, Sawhney R, Wall S, Canto C, et al. Endovascular repair of abdominal aortic aneurysm using a pararenal fenestrated stent-graft. Journal of Endovascular Surgery. 1999;**6**(4):354–358. DOI: 10.1177/152660289900600411

[6] Chuter TA. Fenestrated and branched stent-grafts for thoracoabdominal, pararenal and juxtarenal aortic aneurysm repair. Seminars in Vascular Surgery. 2007;**20** (2):90–96. DOI: 10.1053/j.semvascsurg.2007.04.006

[7] Chuter TA, Gordon RL, Reilly LM, Pak LK, Messina LM. Multi-branched stent-graft for type III thoracoabdominal aortic aneurysm. Journal of Vascular and Interventional Radiology. 2001;**12**(3):391–395. DOI: 10.1016/s1051-0443(07)61924-1

[8] Simons JP, Shue B, Flahive JM, Aiello FA, Steppacher RC, Eaton EA, et al. Trends in use of the only Food and Drug Administration-approved commercially available fenestrated endovascular aneurysm repair device in the United States. Journal of Vascular Surgery. 2017;**65**(6):1687–1697. DOI: 10.1016/j.jvs.2016.10.101

[9] Eleshra A, Hatm M, Spanos K, Panuccio G, Rohlffs F, Debus ES, et al. Early outcomes of t-Branch off-the-shelf multibranched stent graft in urgent and emergent repair of thoracoabdominal aortic aneurysms. Journal of Vascular Surgery. 2022;**75** (2):416–424.e2. DOI: 10.1016/j.jvs.2021.07.237

[10] Oderich GS, Farber MA, Silveira PG, Tadros R, Marin M, Fillinger M, et al. Technical aspects and 30-day outcomes of the prospective early feasibility study of the GORE EXCLUDER Thoracoabdominal Branched Endoprosthesis (TAMBE) to treat pararenal and extent IV thoracoabdominal aortic aneurysms. Journal of Vascular Surgery. 2019;**70** (2):358–368.e6. DOI: 10.1016/j.jvs.2018.10.103

[11] Tran K, Deslarzes-Dubuis C, DeGlise S, Kaladji A, Yang W, Marsden AL, Lee JT. Patient-specific computational flow simulation reveals significant differences in paravisceral

aortic hemodynamics between fenestrated and branched endovascular aneurysm repair. JVS-vascular Science. 2024;**5**:100183. DOI: 10.1016/j.jvssci.2023.100183

[12] Eleshra A, Oderich GS, Spanos K, Panuccio G, Kärkkäinen JM, Tenorio ER, et al. Short-term outcomes of the t-Branch off-the-shelf multibranched stent graft for reintervention after previous infrarenal aortic repair. Journal of Vascular Surgery. 2020;**72**(2):1558–1566. DOI: 10.1016/j.jvs.2020.02.012

[13] Mandelli NCB, Teixeira FF, Barros FCSP, Brunstein LVC. Sliding Rail Technique (Mandelli's), a better method to repair thoracoabdominal aortic aneurysms controlled release fenestrated endoprosthesis. Aorta (Stamford). 2024;**12**(5):126–130. DOI: 10.1055/a-2541-8455

[14] Dias-Neto M, Vacirca A, Huang Y, Baghbani-Oskouei A, Jakimowicz T, Mendes BC, et al. Outcomes of elective and non-elective fenestrated branched endovascular aortic repair for treatment of thoracoabdominal aortic aneurysms. Annals of Surgery. 2023;**278**(4):568–577. DOI: 10.1097/SLA.0000000000005986

[15] Greenberg RK, Lytle B. Endovascular repair of thoracoabdominal aneurysms. Circulation. 2008;**117**(17):2288–2296. DOI: 10.1161/CIRCULATIONAHA.107.716134

[16] Tsilimparis N, Gouveia E Melo R, Tenorio ER, Scali S, Mendes B, Han S, et al. Multicenter study on physician-modified endografts for thoracoabdominal and complex abdominal aortic aneurysm repair. Circulation. 2024;**150**(17):1327–1342. DOI: 10.1161/CIRCULATIONAHA.123.068587

[17] Tan KT, Mafeld SC, Lindsay TF. Endovascular management of unused fenestrations or branches in fenestrated/branched aortic endograft. Journal of Vascular Surgery. 2022;**29**(2):175–180. DOI: 10.1177/15266028211045704

Chapter 5

Clinical and Molecular Risk Factors for Abdominal Aortic Dissection

Mehrdad Sheikhvatan, Hidayet Demir and Mehmet Altuğ Tunçer

Abstract

The aortic wall layers separate in abdominal aortic dissection (AAD), a rare but potentially fatal vascular condition that impairs blood flow, increases the risk of rupture, and causes substantial morbidity and mortality. Combining clinical and molecular viewpoints is necessary to comprehend its pathogenesis. Clinically, AAD is linked to demographic factors like age, sex, and family history, as well as conventional cardiovascular risk factors like smoking, hypertension, atherosclerosis, and connective tissue disorders. Although diagnostic accuracy has increased due to advancements in imaging modalities, timely recognition is still difficult because of its heterogeneous presentation. The aortic wall is weakened, and susceptibility is increased at the molecular level by changes in extracellular matrix remodeling, inflammation, dysregulated signaling of the transforming growth factor-β (TGF-β) pathway, and genetic predispositions involving mutations in genes like FBN1, COL3A1, TGFBR1/2, and ACTA2. In addition to improving risk stratification, the integration of these clinical and molecular correlates directs surveillance procedures, preventative measures, and customized treatment plans. The clinical and molecular determinants of AAD are summarized in this chapter, along with their significance for diagnosis, treatment, and the creation of future focused interventions.

Keywords: abdominal aortic dissection, risk factor, genetics, Risk factor, inflammation

1. Introduction

Abdominal aortic dissection (AAD), is an uncommon yet dangerous type of vascular disease where the aorta tears, creating a new space inside the aorta (false lumen) that causes organs not to get enough blood flow or function. Due to improvements in imaging, increased understanding of patients who present with unusual symptoms, and increased awareness of the specific biological features of AAD, AAD is gaining more clinical attention than in the past when it was thought of as mostly being a part of a larger problem, thoracic aortic disease. An interaction between different types of hemodynamic forces (how blood flows), degenerative changes in the aortic media (the part of the aorta that has muscle), and either genetic changes (mutations in genes) or molecular changes (decreased protein production) are all thought to contribute to the formation of AAD. Scientific research into genomics, proteomics, and molecular imaging has revealed the different mechanisms that contribute to AAD (extracellular matrix remodeling, inflammation, and abnormal smooth muscle cell function) and provides a better understanding of the biology of AAD as well as future directions for treatment. This chapter reviews the most recent clinical evidence regarding the clinical signs of AAD, the methods used to diagnose AAD, and lastly, the biological characteristics of AAD, in order to bridge the gap between clinical observations made at the bedside and the biological research being done on AAD, so as to identify patients who are at highest risk for AAD, identify AAD as soon as possible, and develop treatment strategies for AAD.

2. Overview of abdominal aortic dissection

The separation of the layers of the abdominal aortic wall, which results in a false lumen through which blood can flow, is the hallmark of abdominal aortic dissection (AAD), a potentially fatal vascular condition [1]. This condition is usually caused by an intimal tear that permits blood to pass through the medial layer. This can impair the perfusion of critical abdominal organs and result in life-threatening consequences, such as rupture or end-organ ischemia [2]. AAD carries a considerable risk of morbidity and mortality, especially in patients with comorbidities or delayed diagnosis, even though it is less common than thoracic aortic dissection [3].

Although the prevalence of AAD varies by population, it is typically described as a rare occurrence that accounts for a small portion of all aortic dissections. Although younger patients with connective tissue disorders or genetic predisposition are also at risk, epidemiological studies show a higher prevalence in men and in people 60 years of age and older [4]. Depending on when symptoms start and how the condition develops, AAD can manifest as an acute, sub-acute, or chronic illness. While chronic dissections may remain asymptomatic or present with subtle symptoms, making early detection more difficult, acute cases frequently present with sudden-onset abdominal or back pain, hypotension, or signs of shock [5].

Atherosclerotic disease, connective tissue disorders, and chronic hypertension are among the underlying risk factors that are commonly linked to AAD. The aortic wall is weakened and more vulnerable to dissection as a result of medial degeneration, smooth muscle cell apoptosis, and elastic fiber fragmentation, according to histopathological investigations [6, 7]. Developments in imaging modalities, especially magnetic resonance angiography (MRA) (**Figure 1**) and computed tomography angiography (CTA) (**Figure 2**), have greatly increased diagnostic accuracy, allowing for prompt identification and suitable treatment [8]. Risk assessment, early diagnosis, and treatment decision-making all depend on an understanding of the pathophysiology and clinical manifestation of AAD. The high morbidity and mortality rate linked to this vascular emergency can be significantly decreased by early identification of at-risk individuals, combined with optimal medical and surgical management.

3. Importance of identifying risk factors

Finding the risk factors for AAD is essential for patient outcome optimization, early detection, and prevention. High rates of morbidity and mortality are linked to

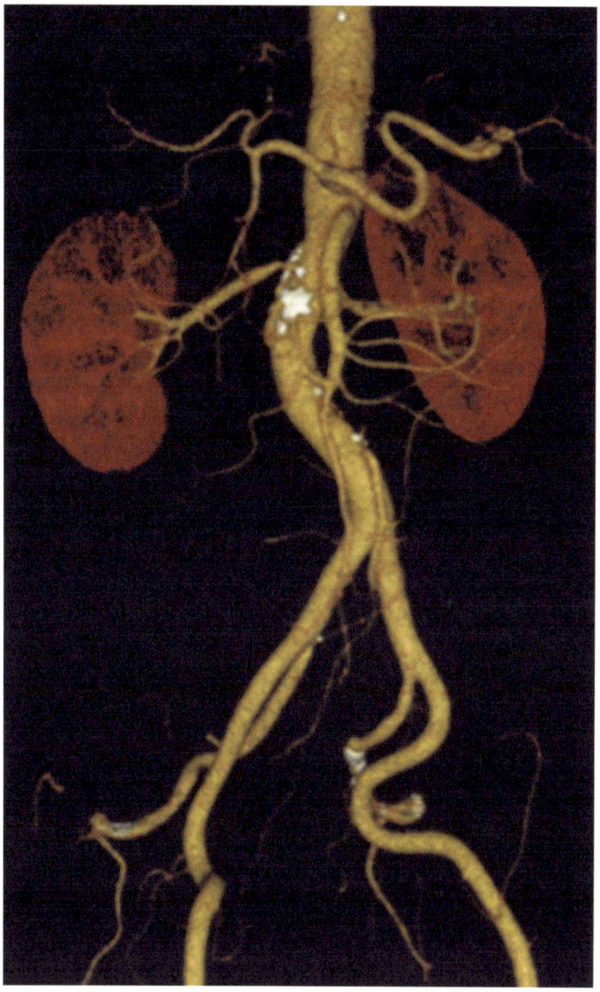

Figure 1.
Three-dimensional contrast-enhanced MR angiography of the abdominal aorta demonstrates an aortic dissection extending into the abdominal segment. The true and false lumens are visualized along the course of the aorta, with a clear depiction of branch vessels, including the renal arteries.

AAD, especially when complications like rupture or organ ischemia arise, or when diagnosis is delayed [9]. Clinicians can stratify patients based on risk and carry out focused interventions by having a thorough understanding of the clinical and molecular factors that predispose people to dissection. Timely monitoring and the implementation of preventive measures, such as strict blood pressure management, lifestyle changes, and, when necessary, elective surgical repair, are made easier by the early identification of high-risk patients [10]. For instance, more frequent imaging surveillance can help identify aortic dilatation or early dissection before catastrophic events occur in patients with known connective tissue disorders or chronic hypertension. Additionally, incorporating genetic and molecular risk factors – like matrix metalloproteinase dysregulation or FBN1 mutations – into risk

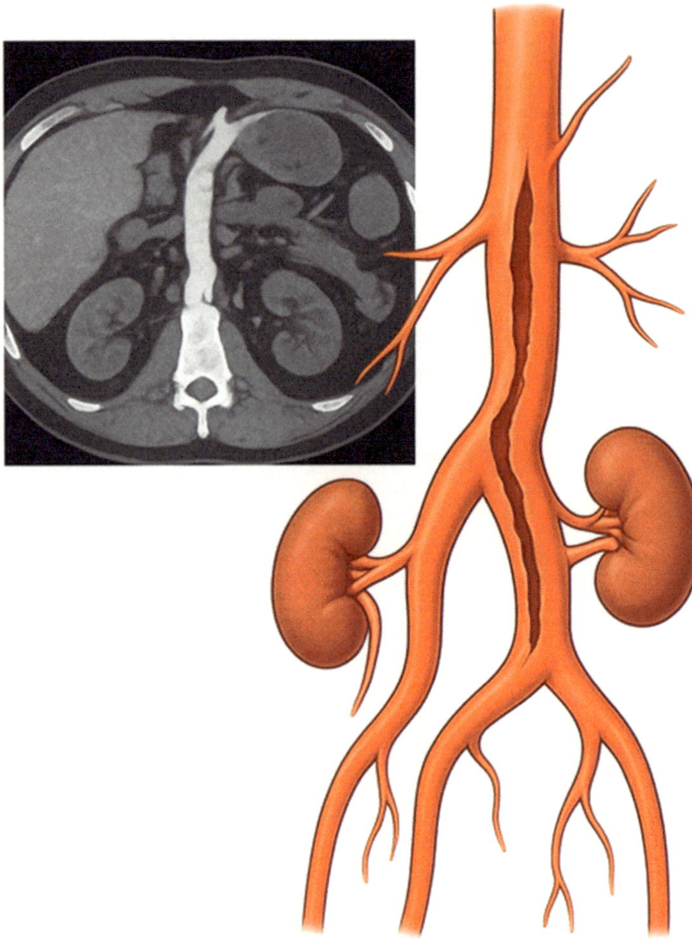

Figure 2.
Computed tomography angiography (CTA) of the abdomen demonstrates an abdominal aortic dissection. The left panel shows an axial CTA slice with contrast enhancement of the true and false lumens within the abdominal aorta.

assessment could make it possible to identify people who seem clinically low-risk but actually have tissue-level vulnerabilities [11, 12].

From the standpoint of clinical management, perioperative and postoperative strategies are informed by knowledge of risk factors. To stop the progression of dissection, high-risk patients might need more stringent blood pressure goals, improved hemodynamic monitoring, or early intervention. Furthermore, risk stratification can help determine when and how to perform endovascular or surgical repair, which will ultimately increase survival rates and lower complications. Lastly, risk factor identification is critical to shared decision-making and patient education. Clinicians can ensure informed consent for invasive procedures and involve patients in preventive measures by communicating individual risk. All things considered, lowering the burden of AAD and enhancing long-term results require a thorough grasp of both clinical and molecular risk factors.

4. Epidemiology and demographics

A relatively rare but clinically significant subset of aortic dissections is AAD. Abdominal involvement presents special diagnostic and treatment challenges, even though thoracic dissections are reported more frequently. With incidence estimates ranging from 2 to 5 cases per 100,000 person-years, epidemiological studies show that AAD makes up a very small portion of all aortic dissections [1, 2, 13]. However, because of asymptomatic or misdiagnosed cases, the actual prevalence might be understated.

AAD primarily affects older adults, with those 60 years of age and older having the highest incidence [4, 14]. Male-to-female ratios have been reported to range from 2:1 to 4:1, indicating that male patients are disproportionately affected. Women with AAD frequently present at an older age and may have a higher perioperative mortality rate despite this male predominance [4, 15]. This is probably due to delayed diagnosis and a higher prevalence of comorbidities.

The afflicted population frequently has risk factors such as hypertension, atherosclerosis, and previous vascular disease [16, 17]. Atypical dissections may also occur in patients with connective tissue disorders, such as Marfan syndrome, Ehlers-Danlos syndrome, and Loeys-Dietz syndrome, who are more vulnerable at an earlier age [18]. A genetic predisposition is suggested by the familial clustering of aortic dissections, and current research attempts to clarify the role of particular gene mutations and polymorphisms in disease susceptibility.

Acute, subacute, and chronic presentations are all possible for AAD. While chronic dissections may remain clinically silent for prolonged periods of time, making epidemiological assessment more difficult, acute presentations are characterized by sudden-onset abdominal or back pain and hemodynamic instability [19]. There have also been reports of geographic variations in incidence, which can be attributed to variations in access to diagnostic imaging, risk factor prevalence, and population demographics [20]. Risk stratification, resource allocation, and the development of preventive measures meant to lower morbidity and mortality all depend on an understanding of the epidemiology and demographic trends of AAD.

5. Clinical risk factors

The onset and course of AAD are significantly influenced by clinical risk factors. Understanding these elements is essential for early identification of high-risk individuals, preventative measures, and customized management plans. Vascular, demographic, genetic, and lifestyle-related factors are the broad categories into which the risk factors can be divided. The most important and common risk factor for AAD is hypertension [21]. Aortic wall mechanical stress caused by persistently high systemic arterial pressure encourages intimal tears and medial degeneration [21]. Vascular remodeling, decreased elasticity, and elevated shear forces are all consequences of both systolic and diastolic hypertension, and they all increase the risk of dissection [21]. The incidence is much higher, and the results are worse for patients with chronic or poorly managed hypertension. Atherosclerotic disease compromises aortic wall integrity through lipid deposition, inflammation, calcification, and weakening of the media. Plaque formation may act as a trigger for intimal tearing and modifies local hemodynamics. The age-related risk of AAD is further explained by the higher prevalence of advanced atherosclerosis in older patients [22].

AAD susceptibility is increased by genetic disorders that affect connective tissue, such as Loeys-Dietz syndrome, Ehlers-Danlos syndrome, and Marfan syndrome. Gene mutations affecting collagen type III, fibrillin-1, or other extracellular matrix components weaken structural support, making aortic walls more likely to dissect even at younger ages. These patients may have recurrent episodes and frequently exhibit early-onset AAD [22]. Degenerative alterations in the aortic media, such as elastin fragmentation, calcification, and loss of smooth muscle cells, are linked to aging and increase susceptibility. With male-to-female ratios ranging from 2:1 to 4:1, men are more likely than women to be impacted. However, women frequently present at later ages and have higher perioperative mortality rates, which may be related to delayed diagnosis [23]. Vascular vulnerability is increased by obesity, smoking, and sedentary lifestyles. Obesity is associated with metabolic syndrome, hypertension, and systemic inflammation, which indirectly raises the risk of dissection, while smoking causes oxidative stress, endothelial dysfunction, and inflammation. Vascular stiffness and poor hemodynamic adaptation are two consequences of physical inactivity [24].

The structural integrity and function of the aorta are impacted by chronic conditions like diabetes mellitus, chronic kidney disease, coronary artery disease, and previous vascular surgery. Diabetes worsens vascular health overall, but paradoxically, it may prevent dissection by making the aorta more rigid. Trauma or previous aortic interventions may change local hemodynamics and make secondary dissections more likely [25, 26]. Dissection in people with underlying vulnerability can be triggered by abrupt spikes in blood pressure, severe physical exertion, or extreme emotional stress. These triggers frequently tip the scales in favor of acute aortic injury by acting on the background of chronic risk factors. A heritable component is suggested by a positive family history of aortic dissection or aneurysm. Genetic variations affecting vascular smooth muscle function or extracellular matrix proteins may increase susceptibility even in the absence of classical connective tissue disorders [3].

When taken together, these clinical risk factors show that chronic vascular stress, genetic predisposition, and environmental or lifestyle factors interact to cause AAD. Clinicians can stratify risk, direct monitoring plans, and carry out focused preventive interventions by thoroughly evaluating these variables, which eventually lower morbidity and mortality.

6. Molecular risk factors

The pathophysiology of AAD is supported by molecular risk factors, which help explain why some people develop dissections even when there are no obvious clinical risk factors. These elements collectively jeopardize the integrity of the aortic wall through structural, cellular, genetic, inflammatory, and biochemical processes.

Various mechanisms and processes have been evaluated and confirmed as responsible for this event, and we will describe each of them.

1. Extracellular matrix (ECM) alterations: Maintaining the elasticity and tensile strength of the aortic wall depends on the ECM, which is mainly

made up of elastin, collagen, proteoglycans, and glycoproteins. ECM homeostasis is disturbed in AAD due to heightened deterioration and inadequate repair. In this process, cystic medial degeneration results from the breakdown of collagen and elastin fibers in the medial layer, caused by the overexpression of Matrix Metalloproteinases (MMPs), particularly MMP-2 and MMP-9. ECM breakdown is further accelerated by decreased expression of MMPs or an imbalance between MMPs and Tissue Inhibitors of Metalloproteinases (TIMPs). Additionally, the aortic wall becomes unstable due to altered proteoglycan synthesis and accumulation, which makes dissection easier [27].

2. Vascular smooth muscle cell (VSMC) dysfunction: Although VSMCs are essential for maintaining the ECM, mediating repair, and offering structural support, their dysfunction greatly accelerates the course of AAD. While phenotypic transition from a contractile to a synthetic state causes aberrant ECM production and the release of inflammatory mediators, apoptosis and senescence result in the loss of VSMCs, which lowers medial tensile strength. Furthermore, VSMC function is further compromised, and aortic wall weakening is encouraged by the dysregulation of important signaling pathways, such as TGF-β, angiotensin II, Notch, and Wnt/β-catenin [28].

3. Inflammation and immune activation: Aortic wall degeneration is primarily caused by inflammation, as increased levels of cytokines like IL-6, TNF-α, and MCP-1 encourage matrix breakdown and VSMC apoptosis. Additionally, immune cells that infiltrate the body, such as neutrophils, T lymphocytes, and macrophages, release reactive oxygen species (ROS) and proteolytic enzymes that further harm the tissue. Even long-term, low-grade vascular inflammation can gradually weaken the aortic wall and make it more vulnerable to dissection [29].

4. Oxidative stress activation: Overproduction of reactive oxygen species (ROS) contributes significantly to the aorta's structural and functional degradation by causing lipid and protein oxidation, which weakens collagen and elastin and reduces vascular elasticity. Furthermore, oxidative stress disrupts nitric oxide signaling, resulting in endothelial dysfunction, increased vascular stiffness, and increased susceptibility to dissection. ROS also increases MMP activity, which accelerates the breakdown of the ECM [30].

5. Genetic and epigenetic factors: Monogenic syndromes like Marfan syndrome, which is caused by mutations in the FBN1 gene, vascular Ehlers-Danlos syndrome, which is linked to mutations in the COL3A1 gene, Loeys-Dietz syndrome, which is linked to mutations in the TGFBR1/2 gene, and ACTA2 mutations, which affect smooth muscle alpha-actin, all significantly increase susceptibility to aortic aneurysm and dissection (AAD). In addition to these syndromic forms, sporadic cases of impaired aortic wall stability are caused by polymorphisms in the genes that control collagen, elastin, and MMPs. Individual susceptibility to AAD is further

shaped by epigenetic mechanisms, which include DNA methylation, histone modifications, and microRNAs like miR-29 and miR-21. These mechanisms are crucial in regulating gene expression linked to vascular smooth muscle cell survival, extracellular matrix turnover, and inflammatory pathways [31, 32].

6. Biochemical and hormonal influences: Aortic pathology is exacerbated by angiotensin II and renin-angiotensin-aldosterone system (RAAS) activation, which encourages oxidative stress, ECM remodeling, and VSMC apoptosis. The observed sex differences in disease incidence may be partially explained by the protective effects of hormones, especially estrogen, on the aortic wall through modulation of ECM metabolism and anti-inflammatory pathways. Apart from MMPs, medial degeneration and aortic wall weakening are also significantly influenced by an imbalance of other proteolytic enzymes, including cathepsins and serine proteases [33, 34].

7. Molecular interactions with clinical risk factors: Clinical risk factors like age-related degeneration, atherosclerosis, and hypertension frequently work in concert with molecular changes. Chronic hypertension, for instance, increases shear stress on an aortic wall that is already weakened by VSMC apoptosis and ECM degradation. The threshold at which mechanical or inflammatory insults cause dissection may also be lowered by genetic mutations [35].

8. Implications for diagnosis and therapy: The development of biomarkers like circulating MMPs, TGF-β, and microRNAs that may be early indicators of aortic vulnerability, the creation of targeted therapies that aim to inhibit MMP activity, modulate TGF-β signaling, or apply antioxidant strategies to stabilize the aortic wall, and the application of personalized medicine approaches that integrate genetic, molecular, and clinical risk profiling to enable individualized monitoring and tailored intervention strategies are just a few of the significant opportunities for improving clinical care that come with an understanding of molecular risk factors.

To sum up, molecular risk factors shed light on the intricate pathophysiology of AAD. Inflammation, oxidative stress, VSMC dysfunction, genetic predisposition, and disruption of ECM integrity all work together to weaken the aortic wall and increase the risk of dissection. Opportunities for early detection, risk assessment, and the creation of focused treatment strategies are presented by developments in our understanding of these pathways.

7. Integrative risk assessment

A thorough strategy that incorporates both clinical and molecular factors is necessary for an accurate risk assessment of AAD. Molecular biomarkers and conventional clinical indicators, by themselves, cannot adequately represent a person's susceptibility; their combination improves prediction accuracy, informs early intervention plans, and directs individualized patient care.

For initial stratification, clinical risk factors – such as age, sex, hypertension, atherosclerosis, and connective tissue disorders – offer a practical and affordable approach [36]. Nonetheless, patients with comparable clinical profiles may show wildly disparate results, indicating the existence of underlying molecular weaknesses. The subclinical processes that directly impair the integrity of the aortic wall are captured by molecular risk factors, which include oxidative stress, inflammation, vascular smooth muscle cell dysfunction, extracellular matrix degradation, and genetic predisposition [37]. A more comprehensive picture of a patient's actual risk can be obtained by combining these layers of data.

In order to enhance risk prediction in aortic dissection, recent research has developed scoring systems and algorithms that combine clinical parameters with molecular and imaging biomarkers. Composite clinical-molecular scores create a dissection risk index by integrating circulating MMP levels or TGF-β activity with variables such as age, hypertension, and family history [38]. To improve the prediction of impending dissection, imaging-molecular techniques combine serum biomarkers or genetic testing with advanced imaging modalities such as CT and MRI, which measure aortic diameter, wall thickness, and intramural hematoma. Additionally, to identify harmful mutations and enhance personalized risk assessment, genetic screening can be combined with clinical evaluation in high-risk groups, particularly those with a family history or connective tissue disorders.

Research indicates that, when it comes to predicting the occurrence and severity of AAD, integrative models perform better than either clinical or molecular markers alone. Higher rates of complications and mortality are seen in patients who are deemed high-risk based on a combined assessment, demonstrating the value of integrative stratification in directing the level of surveillance and treatment choices [39].

By supporting preventive interventions like rigorous blood pressure control, lifestyle changes, and early surgical consultation for those at highest risk, enabling customized surveillance protocols in which high-risk individuals undergo more frequent imaging and laboratory monitoring, and facilitating individualized counseling that communicates risk based on an individual's integrated profile to enhance patient engagement and informed decision-making, integrative risk assessment can govern many aspects of patient care. By combining traditional clinical metrics with omics data (genomics, proteomics, and metabolomics), the field is shifting toward precision medicine approaches. Predictive models could be improved by artificial intelligence and machine learning algorithms, allowing for real-time, personalized risk assessment. To sum up, integrative risk assessment provides a thorough evaluation of AAD susceptibility by combining clinical, molecular, genetic, and imaging data. With the ultimate goal of lowering the morbidity and mortality linked to abdominal aortic dissection, this strategy improves predictive accuracy, directs preventive measures, and facilitates individualized management.

8. Clinical implications

AAD prevention, early detection, management, and follow-up plans are all significantly impacted by an understanding and integration of clinical and molecular risk factors. First, proactive monitoring and intervention are made possible by the identification of high-risk individuals. Imaging modalities like CTA, MRA, or ultrasound can be used to prioritize surveillance for patients with hypertension, atherosclerosis, connective tissue disorders, or pertinent genetic mutations. Before a catastrophic dissection occurs, prompt intervention is possible when aortic wall abnormalities like dilatation, intramural hematoma, or focal medial degeneration are identified early [40]. Second, the frequency and severity of follow-up are determined by integrative risk assessment. While low-risk individuals can adhere to standard surveillance procedures, high-risk patients might need more frequent imaging and biomarker monitoring. Personalized follow-up plans guarantee early detection in susceptible groups while minimizing unnecessary testing. Third, preventive measures are guided by clinical and molecular risk profiles. Stress on the aortic wall can be reduced by aggressive blood pressure control, lifestyle changes (such as quitting smoking, controlling weight, and exercising), and managing comorbid conditions like diabetes or renal disease [41]. As precision medicine advances, new therapeutic approaches that target these pathways may become relevant for patients with high molecular risk, such as elevated MMPs, TGF-β dysregulation, or pathogenic gene variants. To stop progression or rupture, high-risk patients may benefit from elective surgery or endovascular repair [42]. Fourth, informed decision-making and patient education are improved by integrative risk assessment. Clinicians can discuss the possibility of complications, the potential advantages of interventions, and lifestyle changes by providing patients with personalized risk profiles. This method strengthens shared decision-making and increases adherence to preventive measures. Finally, better healthcare resource allocation, high-risk patient prioritization, and targeted clinical trial design are made possible by the identification of risk factors at both the clinical and molecular levels. Risk stratification will be improved, and outcomes will be enhanced by ongoing research into biomarkers, genetic screening, and molecular therapies. Ultimately, early detection, risk-based monitoring, focused interventions, and individualized counseling are all influenced by knowledge of the clinical and molecular risk factors for AAD. By implementing these strategies, one can lower morbidity and mortality, maximize resource use, and encourage the advancement of precision medicine techniques for AAD.

9. Future directions

Although we now have a much better understanding of AAD, there are still many opportunities to enhance therapeutic intervention, risk assessment, and early detection. In order to lower the high morbidity and mortality linked to this condition, future research is probably going to concentrate on creating targeted interventions and incorporating clinical, molecular, genetic, and imaging data into predictive models. The goal of ongoing research is to find new genetic variations, epigenetic changes, and molecular biomarkers that make people more susceptible to AAD. Transcriptomics, proteomics, and whole-genome sequencing techniques may reveal hitherto unknown pathways connected to inflammation, vascular smooth muscle cell dysfunction, and extracellular matrix remodeling. These findings may help develop early intervention plans and individualized risk assessments. Circulating biomarkers, including MMPs, transforming growth factor-beta (TGF-β), and microRNAs (e.g., miR-29, miR-21), are being investigated for their potential to predict imminent dissection or disease progression. Early diagnosis, risk-guided treatment planning, and non-invasive monitoring may all be made possible by the validation of these biomarkers. Also, precision medicine in AAD may be possible by combining cutting-edge computational models with clinical, molecular, and genetic data. The accuracy of risk prediction may be increased by machine learning and artificial intelligence algorithms, enabling personalized surgical planning, medical therapy, and surveillance schedules. In addition, a growing area of interest is targeted therapies that target the molecular mechanisms underlying AAD. Strategies like MMP inhibitors, TGF-β modulators, antioxidant treatments, and substances that support the survival of vascular smooth muscle cells may be used in addition to standard medical and surgical procedures. To prove safety and efficacy, preclinical research and early-stage clinical trials are necessary. In addition, aortic wall biomechanics and flow patterns can be thoroughly evaluated using high-resolution imaging techniques, such as intravascular ultrasound and 4D-flow MRI. The early detection of aortic wall instability prior to overt dissection may be improved by combining these imaging insights with molecular biomarkers.

Author details

Mehrdad Sheikhvatan*, Hidayet Demir and Mehmet Altuğ Tunçer
Cardiovascular Surgery Research Center, Istanbul Okan University, Istanbul, Turkey

*Address all correspondence to: med.msv@gmail.com

References

[1] Wu J, Zafar M, Qiu J, Huang Y, Chen Y, Yu C, Elefteriades JA. A systematic review and meta-analysis of isolated abdominal aortic dissection. Journal of Vascular Surgery. 2019;**70**(6):2046–2053.e6

[2] Lech C, Swaminathan A. Abdominal aortic emergencies. Emergency Medicine Clinics of North America. 2017;**35**(4):847–867

[3] Sherifova S, Holzapfel GA. Biomechanics of aortic wall failure with a focus on dissection and aneurysm: A review. Acta Biomaterialia. 2019;**99**:1–17

[4] Vermeersch N, Hendriks JM, Lauwers P, Salgado R, Van Schil PE. Aortic dissection limited to abdominal aorta: An underrecognized entity ? Acta Chirurgica Belgica. 2015;**115**(4):293–298

[5] Li Y, Jiao Y, Li W, He C, Zhang H, Zhang T. Management of isolated abdominal aortic dissection: Indications and strategies for treatment. Annals of Vascular Surgery. 2024;**99**:117–124

[6] Sen I, D'Oria M, Weiss S, Bower TC, Oderich GS, Kalra M, Colglazier J, DeMartino RR. Incidence and natural history of isolated abdominal aortic dissection: A population-based assessment from 1995 to 2015. Journal of Vascular Surgery. 2021;**73**(4):1198–1204.e1

[7] Jonker FH, Schlösser FJ, Moll FL, Muhs BE. Dissection of the abdominal aorta. Current evidence and implications for treatment strategies: A review and meta-analysis of 92 patients. Journal of Endovascular Therapy. 2009;**16**(1):71–80

[8] Martufi G, Gasser TC, Appoo JJ, Di Martino ES. Mechano-biology in the thoracic aortic aneurysm: A review and case study. Biomechanics and Modeling in Mechanobiology. 2014;**13**(5):917–928

[9] Baumann F, Makaloski V, Diehm N. Aortic aneurysms and aortic dissection: Epidemiology, pathophysiology and diagnostics. Der Internist. 2013;**54**(5):535–542

[10] Huckaby LV, Leshnower BG. Sex and gender differences in aortic disease. US Cardiology. 2023;**17**:e14

[11] DiLosa K, Brittenham G, Pozolo C, Hedayati N, Kwong M, Maximus S, Humphries M. Evaluating growth patterns of abdominal aortic aneurysms among women. Journal of Vascular Surgery. 2024;**80**(1):107–113

[12] Patel K, Zafar MA, Ziganshin BA, Elefteriades JA. Diabetes mellitus: Is it protective against aneurysm? A narrative review. Cardiology. 2018;**141**(2):107–122

[13] Marcaccio CL, O'Donnell TFX, Dansey KD, Patel PB, Hughes K, Lo RC, Zettervall SL, Schermerhorn ML. Disparities in reporting and representation by sex, race, and ethnicity in endovascular aortic device trials. Journal of Vascular Surgery. 2022;**76**(5):1244–1252.e2

[14] Lidén K, Jonsson M, Stackelberg O, Steuer J, Krasun M, Smedberg C. Acute symptomatic isolated abdominal aortic dissection – Clinical characteristics, outcome, and sex differences. Annals of Vascular Surgery. 2024;**106**:61–70

[15] Wu S, Cao C, Lun Y, Jiang H, Wang S, He Y, Sun J, Li X, He Y, Huang Y, Chen W, Xin S, Zhang J. Age-related differences in acute aortic dissection. Journal of Vascular Surgery. 2022;**75**(2):473–483.e4

[16] Vogt BA, Birk PE, Panzarino V, Hite SH, Kashtan CE. Aortic dissection in young patients with chronic hypertension. American Journal of Kidney Diseases. 1999;**33**(2):374–378

[17] Sato M, Imai A, Sakamoto H, Sasaki A, Watanabe Y, Jikuya T. Abdominal aortic disease caused by penetrating atherosclerotic ulcers. Annals of Vascular Diseases. 2012;**5**(1):8–14

[18] Shalhub S, Byers PH, Hicks KL, Charlton-Ouw K, Zarkowsky D, Coleman DM, Davis FM, Regalado ES, De Caridi G, Weaver KN, Miller EM, Schermerhorn ML, Shean K, Oderich G, Ribeiro M, Nishikawa C, Behrendt CA, Debus ES, von Kodolitsch Y, Powell RJ, Pepin M, Milewicz DM, Lawrence PF, Woo K. A multi-institutional experience in the aortic and arterial pathology in individuals with genetically confirmed vascular Ehlers-Danlos syndrome. Journal of Vascular Surgery. 2019;**70**(5):1543–1554

[19] Mukherjee D, Eagle KA. Aortic dissection—An update. Current Problems in Cardiology. 2005;**30**(6):287–325

[20] Zhao Z, Liu J, Liu Y, Huang K, Wang M, Wu R, Hu Z, Yao C, Li Z, Chang G. Clinical characteristics and therapeutic strategy for patients with spontaneous isolated abdominal aortic dissection. Frontiers in Cardiovascular Medicine. 2023;**10**:1214377

[21] Giannakoulas G, Giannoglou G, Soulis J, Farmakis T, Papadopoulou S, Parcharidis G, Louridas G. A computational model to predict aortic wall stresses in patients with systolic arterial hypertension. Medical Hypotheses. 2005;**65**(6):1191–1195

[22] Kuhlencordt PJ, Gyurko R, Han F, Scherrer-Crosbie M, Aretz TH, Hajjar R, Picard MH, Huang PL. Accelerated atherosclerosis, aortic aneurysm formation, and ischemic heart disease in apolipoprotein E/endothelial nitric oxide synthase double-knockout mice. Circulation. 2001;**104**(4):448–454

[23] Carbone RG, Monselise A, Puppo F. Marfan syndrome and aortic involvement: A narrative review. European Review for Medical and Pharmacological Sciences. 2023;**27**(17):8218–8224

[24] Skotsimara G, Antonopoulos A, Oikonomou E, Papastamos C, Siasos G, Tousoulis D. Aortic wall inflammation in the pathogenesis, diagnosis and treatment of aortic aneurysms. Inflammation. 2022;**45**(3):965–976

[25] Berthet J-P, Marty-Ané C-H, Veerapen R, Picard E, Mary H, Alric P. Dissection of the abdominal aorta in blunt trauma: Endovascular or conventional surgical management? Journal of Vascular Surgery. 2003;**38**(5):997–1003

[26] Hundersmarck D, Toorop RJ. Aortoiliac dissection after blunt abdominal trauma. European Journal of Vascular and Endovascular Surgery. 2018;**55**(5):613

[27] Ishii T, Asuwa N. Collagen and elastin degradation by matrix metalloproteinases and tissue inhibitors

of matrix metalloproteinase in aortic dissection. Human Pathology. 2000;**31** (6):640–646

[28] Rombouts KB, van Merrienboer Tar, Ket JCF, Bogunovic JCF, van der Velden J, Yeung KK. The role of vascular smooth muscle cells in the development of aortic aneurysms and dissections. European Journal of Clinical Investigation. 2022;**52**(4):e13697

[29] Tsilimigras DI, Sigala F, Karaolanis G, Ntanasis-Stathopoulos I, Spartalis E, Spartalis M, Patelis N, Papalampros A, Long C, Moris D. Cytokines as biomarkers of inflammatory response after open versus endovascular repair of abdominal aortic aneurysms: A systematic review. Acta Pharmacologica Sinica. 2018;**39** (7):1164–1175

[30] Zhang L, Wang C, Xi Z, Li D, Xu Z. Mercaptoethanol protects the aorta from dissection by inhibiting oxidative stress, inflammation, and extracellular matrix degeneration in a mouse model. Medical Science Monitor. 2018;**24**: 1802–1812

[31] Kumar S, Boon RA, Maegdefessel L, Dimmeler S, Jo H. Role of noncoding RNAs in the pathogenesis of abdominal aortic aneurysm. Circulation Research. 2019;**124**(4): 619–630

[32] Milewicz DM. MicroRNAs, fibrotic remodeling, and aortic aneurysms. Journal of Clinical Investigation. 2012;**122**(2):490–493

[33] Luo W, Wang Y, Zhang L, Ren P, Zhang C, Li Y, Azares AR, Zhang M, Guo J, Ghaghada KB, Starosolski ZA, Rajapakshe K, Coarfa C, Li Y, Chen R, Fujiwara K, Abe JI, Coselli JS, Milewicz DM, LeMaire SA, Shen YH. Critical Role of Cytosolic DNA and Its Sensing Adaptor STING in Aortic Degeneration, Dissection, and Rupture. Circulation. 2020;**141**(1):42–66

[34] Li T, Lv Z, Jing JJ, Yang J, Yuan Y. Matrix metalloproteinase family polymorphisms and the risk of aortic aneurysmal diseases: A systematic review and meta-analysis. Clinical Genetics. 2018;**93**(1):15–32

[35] Zhou H, Wang Z. Aortic dissection and vascular smooth muscle cell apoptosis: In-depth exploration of their relationship and potential therapeutic strategies. Zhonghua Wei Zhong Bing Ji Jiu Yi Xue. 2025;**37**(3):225–231

[36] Nazerian P, Mueller C, Soeiro AM, Leidel BA, Salvadeo SAT, Giachino F, Vanni S, Grimm K, Mt Jr O, Pivetta E, Lupia E, Grifoni S, Morello F. ADvISED Investigators. Diagnostic Accuracy of the Aortic Dissection Detection Risk Score Plus D-Dimer for Acute Aortic Syndromes: The ADvISED Prospective Multicenter Study. Circulation. 2018;**137**(3):250–258

[37] Landenhed M, Engström G, Gottsäter A, Caulfield MP, Hedblad B, Newton-Cheh C, Melander O, Smith JG. Risk profiles for aortic dissection and ruptured or surgically treated aneurysms: A prospective cohort study. Journal of the American Heart Association. 2015;**4**(1):12–16

[38] Erbel R, Aboyans V, Boileau C, Bossone E, Bartolomeo RD, Eggebrecht H, Evangelista A, Falk V, Frank H, Gaemperli O, Grabenwöger M, Haverich A, Iung B, Manolis AJ, Meijboom F, Nienaber CA, Roffi M, Rousseau H, Sechtem U, Sirnes PA, Allmen RS, Vrints CJ; ESC Committee for Practice Guidelines. 2014 ESC Guidelines on the diagnosis and

treatment of aortic diseases: Document covering acute and chronic aortic diseases of the thoracic and abdominal aorta of the adult. The Task Force for the Diagnosis and Treatment of Aortic Diseases of the European Society of Cardiology (ESC). European Heart Journal. 2014;**35**(41):2873–2926

[39] Trimarchi S, Tsai T, Eagle KA, Isselbacher EM, Froehlich J, Cooper JV, Rampoldi V, GR Jr U. International Registry of Acute Aortic Dissection (IRAD) investigators. Acute abdominal aortic dissection: Insight from the International Registry of Acute Aortic Dissection (IRAD). Journal of Vascular Surgery. 2007;**46**(5):913–919

[40] Kouvelos GN, Vourliotakis G, Arnaoutoglou E, Papa N, Avgos S, Peroulis M, Papadopoulos G, Matsagkas MI. Endovascular treatment for isolated acute abdominal aortic dissection. Journal of Vascular Surgery. 2013;**58**(6):1505–1511

[41] Hu SS. Aortic disease and peripheral artery disease. Journal of Geriatric Cardiology. 2024;**21**(10): 931–943

[42] Michel JB, Jondeau G, Milewicz DM. From genetics to response to injury: Vascular smooth muscle cells in aneurysms and dissections of the ascending aorta. Cardiovascular Research. 2018;**114** (4):578–589

Chapter 6

Hybrid Approaches for Complex Abdominal Aortic Aneurysms: A Literature Review of Open and Endovascular Combined Techniques

Ersin Ozer

Abstract

Treatment of complex abdominal aortic aneurysms (AAAs), particularly thoracoabdominal aortic aneurysms (TAAAs), remains a significant surgical challenge associated with high morbidity and mortality. While conventional open surgical repair (OSR) has long been the gold standard, its invasiveness has prompted the development of less invasive alternatives. Endovascular aneurysm repair (EVAR) has revolutionized AAA treatment but is often limited by hostile anatomy, such as severe iliac artery calcification, extensive dissections, or inadequate landing zones, especially in cases involving visceral arteries. Hybrid repair, which combines open surgical debranching of visceral and renal arteries with endovascular stent-grafting, has emerged as a viable alternative for high-risk patients or those with anatomies unsuitable for standard OSR or total endovascular repair. This chapter provides a comprehensive literature review of hybrid techniques for complex AAAs. It examines patient selection criteria, procedural variations including staged versus single-stage repairs, the "funnel" and "chunnel" techniques, and strategies for managing prior aortic repairs, and discusses outcomes related to mortality, morbidity, spinal cord ischemia, renal failure, and long-term graft patency. Furthermore, it addresses special patient populations, such as those with genetic aortopathies or ruptured aneurysms, and contextualizes the role of hybrid procedures in an era of advancing endovascular technologies. By synthesizing evidence from case reports, series, and comparative studies, this review outlines the current status, technical feasibility, and clinical efficacy of hybrid approaches in the management of complex aortic disease.

Keywords: abdominal aortic aneurysm, hybrid surgical procedures, endovascular aneurysm repair, visceral debranching, thoracoabdominal aortic aneurysm, complex aortic disease

1. Introduction

1.1 Pathophysiology and epidemiology of abdominal aortic aneurysm

An abdominal aortic aneurysm (AAA) is a localized dilatation of the abdominal aorta, most commonly occurring in the infrarenal segment, defined as an aortic diameter greater than 3 cm or 1.5 times the normal vessel diameter [1]. The prevalence of this condition is significantly influenced by age and gender, rising from 1.3% in men aged 55–64 to 9.1% in those aged 65–74, and reaching as high as 22% in men over 85 [2]. While less common in women, the risk of rupture is four times higher in females for any given aneurysm diameter [3]. The natural history of AAA is characterized by progressive expansion, and the risk of rupture increases exponentially with aneurysm size, rising from approximately 1% per year for aneurysms under 5.5 cm to 10% per year for those between 5.5 and 6.9 cm. Given that a ruptured AAA (rAAA) is a catastrophic event with a mortality rate exceeding 80%, timely intervention is critical [1, 2].

The pathophysiology of AAA is a complex process distinct from simple atherosclerosis [3]. It is driven by a cascade of chronic inflammation, proteolytic degradation of the extracellular matrix (primarily elastin and collagen), and depletion of vascular smooth muscle cells (VSMCs) [1, 4]. This process leads to a progressive weakening and structural failure of the aortic wall. Key risk factors that initiate or accelerate these pathological changes include advanced age, male sex, a history of smoking, hypertension, dyslipidemia, and a family history of AAA [3]. Of these, cigarette smoking is the most significant modifiable risk factor, being more strongly associated with AAA than with coronary or cerebrovascular disease.

1.2 The gold standard and its challenges: Conventional open surgical repair

Since its first successful report in 1951, open surgical repair (OSR) has been the established gold standard for treating large AAAs [2, 5]. The procedure involves a major laparotomy with a transperitoneal or retroperitoneal approach, followed by replacement of the aneurysmal segment with a durable synthetic graft. In high-volume centers, elective OSR for infrarenal AAA can be performed with excellent outcomes, with 30-day mortality rates reported as low as 2.5% [5]. However, OSR is a highly invasive procedure associated with significant physiological stress and considerable perioperative morbidity and mortality [6]. In the emergency setting of a ruptured AAA, the 30-day mortality for OSR remains high, approaching 30%, even in specialized centers [5]. The invasiveness of the procedure is magnified in the context of more extensive thoracoabdominal aortic aneurysms (TAAAs), which require thoracotomy, aortic cross-clamping above the visceral vessels, and extracorporeal circulation, leading to higher rates of complications such as spinal cord ischemia (SCI), renal failure, and respiratory failure.

1.3 The endovascular revolution: The rise and limitations of endovascular aneurysm repair

The introduction of endovascular aneurysm repair (EVAR) in the 1990s represented a paradigm shift in AAA management [3, 7]. This minimally invasive technique involves the percutaneous deployment of a stent-graft to exclude the aneurysm sac from circulation, thereby avoiding a major abdominal incision [2]. Large randomized controlled trials (EVAR-1, DREAM, OVER) demonstrated a significant short-term survival benefit for EVAR over OSR, with lower 30-day morbidity and mortality rates [2, 5]. Consequently, EVAR quickly became the first-line treatment for the majority of patients with anatomically suitable infrarenal AAAs [2].

However, the initial enthusiasm for EVAR has been tempered by concerns regarding its long-term durability [5]. The early survival benefit diminishes over time, and EVAR is associated with a higher rate of late complications, including endoleaks, stent-graft migration, and component separation, which often necessitate secondary interventions [2]. The most significant limitation of standard EVAR, however, is its dependence on favorable aortoiliac anatomy [2, 8]. A significant proportion of patients, estimated to be between 31% and 42% in some studies, do not meet the strict anatomical criteria outlined in the instructions for use (IFU) for commercially available endografts [9].

1.4 Defining the "complex" aneurysm: Anatomical and clinical hostility

The term "complex AAA" refers to a heterogeneous group of aneurysms that are not amenable to standard infrarenal EVAR due to hostile anatomical features. These features compromise the ability to achieve a secure and durable seal, prevent device delivery, or maintain perfusion to vital branch arteries. Key anatomical challenges include:

- **Hostile proximal neck:** The proximal landing zone may be too short (<10–15 mm), severely angulated, conical (reverse tapered), or excessively wide (>32 mm), all of which are strong predictors of type Ia endoleak and long-term failure [8, 10, 11].

- **Severe iliac artery disease:** Heavy circumferential calcification can make iliac arteries unsuitable for clamping during OSR and poses a risk of rupture during endograft delivery [8]. Similarly, severe stenosis or occlusion of the iliac arteries can prevent the passage of large-profile delivery systems required for EVAR [12].

- **Involvement of visceral arteries:** The aneurysm may extend proximally to involve the renal, superior mesenteric, or celiac arteries. These are classified as juxtarenal, pararenal, or TAAAs and represent the most challenging subset of complex aortic disease [11,13].

These anatomical complexities, often compounded by significant patient comorbidities, create a cohort of patients for whom neither standard OSR nor standard EVAR is an ideal solution, necessitating alternative treatment strategies.

1.5 The genesis of hybrid repair: Bridging the gap between open and endovascular techniques

Hybrid repair emerged in the late 1990s as a novel solution to bridge the gap between the durability of open surgery and the reduced invasiveness of endovascular techniques [13, 14]. The core philosophy of the hybrid approach is to combine a targeted open surgical procedure with an endovascular stent-graft placement to treat complex aortic pathologies [15, 16]. For complex AAAs, this most often involves an open surgical component to revascularize the visceral and renal arteries through bypass grafts (debranching), thereby creating a new, disease-free landing zone for the subsequent endovascular exclusion of the aneurysm sac with a stent graft [13].

This strategy was developed as a therapeutic alternative for high-risk patients who were considered unfit for the rigors of conventional TAAA repair [17]. By avoiding a thoracotomy, supraceliac aortic clamping, and prolonged single-lung ventilation, the hybrid approach aims to reduce major perioperative complications while still providing a definitive and durable repair [13]. Over the past two decades, the application of hybrid techniques has expanded significantly, with numerous variations developed to address a wide array of anatomical challenges. This chapter will provide a comprehensive review of the contemporary literature on hybrid repair for complex AAAs, detailing patient selection criteria, procedural techniques, clinical outcomes, and the evolving role of this approach in modern vascular surgery.

2. Principles and patient selection for hybrid aortic surgery

The paradigm of hybrid aortic surgery is built upon a foundation of strategic problem-solving for patients who fall into the treatment gap between conventional open and total endovascular repairs. The procedure is not a universal replacement for either but serves as a critical alternative tailored to a specific subset of patients with high surgical risk and hostile anatomy. Its principles are centered on minimizing physiological insult while ensuring a durable and effective aneurysm exclusion.

2.1 Fundamental rationale: Preserving visceral perfusion and creating a viable landing zone

The core tenet of hybrid repair for complex AAAs and TAAAs is the surgical creation of a new, healthy landing zone to facilitate a stable endovascular seal, while simultaneously ensuring uninterrupted perfusion to the vital visceral and renal arteries. In complex aneurysms, particularly those extending into the pararenal or thoracoabdominal segments, the native aorta at the level of the visceral vessels is diseased and unsuitable for anchoring an endograft. The hybrid approach circumvents this problem by surgically rerouting the circulation to the celiac, superior mesenteric, and renal arteries via prosthetic bypass grafts – a process known as "debranching". This open surgical component effectively relocates the origins of these critical vessels to a healthy inflow source, such as the infrarenal aorta or the iliac arteries. Once the visceral segment of the aorta is "decommissioned," it becomes a passive conduit, allowing for the deployment of a thoracic endograft (TEVAR) to bridge the aneurysmal aorta and achieve exclusion. This strategy obviates the need for a thoracotomy, supraceliac aortic clamping, and extracorporeal circulation, which are major sources of morbidity in conventional open TAAA repair [18].

2.2 Identifying the ideal candidate: A risk–benefit analysis

The decision to proceed with a hybrid repair is a multifactorial one, balancing the patient's physiological resilience against their specific anatomical challenges. The ideal candidate is often one for whom the risks of OSR are prohibitive, yet the anatomy is too complex for a standard or even an advanced total endovascular approach [18].

2.2.1 High-risk patients unsuitable for open repair

Hybrid procedures were initially developed and continue to be primarily indicated for patients considered "high-risk" or unfit for conventional open surgery. This risk is often quantified using the American Society of Anesthesiologists (ASA) physical status classification, with patients in classes 3 and 4 being common candidates for hybrid repair. Significant comorbidities that favor a less invasive approach include severe coronary artery disease, congestive heart failure, significant chronic obstructive pulmonary disease (COPD), and advanced age. In one large 10-year series, the mean patient age was 72.7 years, with 68% of patients being over 70. The presence of a "hostile abdomen" from multiple previous laparotomies, which would make open dissection hazardous, also weighs in favor of a hybrid strategy. Furthermore, patients with a limited life expectancy, such as those with active malignancy, may be offered a hybrid repair as a palliative measure to prevent imminent rupture without subjecting them to the long recovery of a major open operation [18].

2.2.2 Anatomical unsuitability for total endovascular repair

While fenestrated and branched EVAR (F/B-EVAR) has become a primary treatment for complex aneurysms, it is not universally applicable. Hybrid repair serves as a crucial alternative when total endovascular approaches are contraindicated by anatomical constraints. Such constraints include:

- **Inadequate access vessels:** Severe stenosis, calcification, tortuosity, or occlusion of the femoral or iliac arteries can prevent the safe passage of the large-profile delivery systems required for F/B-EVAR. Atrophic iliac arteries, such as those seen in patients with post-poliomyelitis sequelae, can also preclude an endovascular-first approach.

- **Unfavorable target vessel anatomy:** Visceral arteries with severe ostial stenosis, calcification, sharp downward-facing angulation, or early bifurcation can make catheterization and stenting during F/B-EVAR technically challenging or impossible.

- **Complex aortic anatomy:** Extreme aortic tortuosity or complex anatomy associated with chronic dissection can make the precise deployment of custom fenestrated/branched devices difficult.

- **Urgency:** In urgent or ruptured scenarios, the six- to eight-week manufacturing time for a custom F/B-EVAR device is prohibitive, making an off-the-shelf hybrid approach a more viable and immediate option [18].

2.3 The role of advanced imaging: Hybrid operating rooms and preoperative planning

The execution of complex hybrid procedures is heavily reliant on high-quality, real-time imaging. The advent of the hybrid operating room – a sterile surgical suite equipped with a fixed, high-power angiography C-arm – has been a significant enabler for these techniques. Compared to a standard operating room with a mobile C-arm, a hybrid OSR offers superior image quality and advanced applications like three-dimensional (3D) rotational angiography, cone-beam computed tomography (CBCT), and image fusion with preoperative CT scans. These tools are invaluable for precise guidewire navigation, accurate deployment of endografts, and immediate detection of complications like endoleaks. Studies have shown that while procedural times may not differ, the use of a hybrid OSR for complex endovascular procedures can significantly reduce the required volume of nephrotoxic contrast medium, which is a critical benefit for a patient population that often has pre-existing renal insufficiency. Furthermore, in urgent settings, the "Hybrid Emergency Room" concept integrates diagnostic CT, angiography, and surgical capabilities into a single space, drastically reducing the "door-to-intervention" time for patients with ruptured aneurysms by eliminating inter-departmental transfers.

Meticulous preoperative planning using high-resolution, thin-slice (e.g., 1 mm) CTA is mandatory. Advanced 3D workstation software is used to perform centerline analysis, measure precise distances and diameters, and map the clock positions of visceral vessel ostia, which is essential for planning both the open debranching and the subsequent endovascular exclusion [18].

3. Core surgical component: Visceral and renal debranching techniques

The open surgical component is the cornerstone of a hybrid aortic repair, designed to meticulously re-route blood flow to the vital visceral and renal arteries before the diseased aortic segment is excluded endovascularly. This "debranching" procedure is a major abdominal operation that requires a deep understanding of retroperitoneal anatomy and versatile vascular anastomotic skills. The approach has evolved from traditional hand-sewn techniques to include innovative, time-saving strategies that minimize organ ischemia.

3.1 Standard retrograde revascularization from aortoiliac inflow

The most common method for visceral debranching is retrograde revascularization, where the inflow for the new bypass grafts originates from a source distal to the aneurysm [2]. This approach is typically performed through a transperitoneal midline laparotomy, which provides wide exposure of the abdominal aorta and its branches [19]. The inflow is most frequently established from the common or external iliac arteries, which are chosen based on the extent of the native disease and the absence of severe calcification or occlusion. In patients with heavily diseased iliac arteries or a prior history of abdominal aortic replacement, the existing infrarenal aortic graft or a healthy segment of the infrarenal aorta itself can serve as a robust inflow source [2].

The fundamental concept involves anastomosing a primary prosthetic graft to the chosen inflow vessel. From this primary graft, individual bypasses are then constructed to supply the celiac artery, superior mesenteric artery (SMA), and both renal arteries [2, 19]. This re-plumbing of the visceral circulation effectively moves the functional origin of these critical arteries to a distal, healthy segment, thereby creating a long, uninterrupted landing zone in the native aorta for subsequent endograft deployment [14].

3.2 Procedural nuances: Graft configuration and anastomotic strategies

The technical execution of visceral debranching involves several key decisions regarding graft configuration and anastomotic technique. Surgeons may use customized Y-grafts, separate bypass grafts, or commercially available multi-branched prostheses to fashion the revascularization [13]. A common configuration involves anastomosing a primary bifurcated graft (e.g., 18 × 9 mm) to the inflow source, followed by the attachment of pre-sewn smaller bifurcated or quadrifurcated grafts (e.g., the "InterGard Quattro" graft) to the limbs of this primary graft, from which the individual visceral bypasses originate [6, 19]. This modular approach allows for flexibility in tailoring the geometry of the bypasses to the patient's specific anatomy.

The anastomoses to the target vessels are performed in either an end-to-end or end-to-side manner. For the renal arteries, an end-to-end anastomosis is often preferred after the native artery is transected, which can provide favorable geometry and reduce the risk of kinking. For the celiac trunk and SMA, which have a broader and more complex collateral network, an end-to-side anastomosis is typically performed to preserve any existing native flow during the construction of the bypass [19]. To avoid compression, the graft to the celiac artery is often tunneled retro-pancreatically [6, 13]. A critical step in the procedure is the ligation or embolization of the native visceral artery origins after the bypasses are completed. This is essential to prevent retrograde perfusion of the aneurysm sac from these vessels after the endograft is deployed, which would result in a persistent type II endoleak and potential treatment failure [14].

3.3 Innovations in debranching: Sutureless techniques and the "chunnel" approach

Recognizing the morbidity associated with prolonged organ ischemia and extensive dissection, innovative techniques have been developed to streamline the debranching process.

3.3.1 Sutureless anastomosis with covered stents

One of the most significant challenges during renal artery revascularization is the duration of warm ischemia, which traditionally lasts 10–25 minutes for a hand-sewn anastomosis and can contribute to postoperative acute kidney injury [13]. To address this, a "sutureless" or telescoping anastomosis using a covered stent-graft (e.g., GORE® VIABAHN®) has been described [9, 13]. In this technique, a bypass graft is sutured to the main inflow graft. The Viabahn device is then advanced through the bypass graft and deployed directly into the target renal artery through a small arteriotomy. The stent graft creates a seal against the arterial wall without the need for sutures, reducing the renal warm ischemia time to as little as two minutes. This technique has proven to be a workable and effective option, especially in deep and difficult-to-access renal arteries [13].

3.3.2 The "Chunnel debranching" technique

To further minimize the invasiveness of visceral debranching, particularly in patients with a hostile abdomen from prior surgeries, the novel "Chunnel debranching" technique has been developed. This procedure is performed through a retroperitoneal approach, avoiding a full laparotomy and the need for deep dissection around vital abdominal organs. The technique involves first anastomosing a prosthetic graft onto the exposed wall of the aneurysm itself using an inclusion technique. A covered stent (Viabahn) is then guided by fluoroscopy and epi-aortic ultrasound through this external graft, puncturing the aortic wall and traversing the aneurysm sac to be deployed directly into the ostium of the target visceral artery [13]. This creates a "channel" or "tunnel" from the bypass graft to the visceral artery through the aneurysm. This innovative approach significantly reduces dissection and manipulation of intraperitoneal structures, offering a potentially safer option for reoperative surgery or for patients with severe intra-abdominal adhesions.
A schematic overview of the Chunnel debranching technique, illustrating the creation of Viabahn stent channels from the iliac inflow graft to the visceral arteries, is presented in **Figure 1**.

4. Spectrum of hybrid procedures for complex aortoiliac disease

The flexibility of the hybrid paradigm allows for a wide spectrum of procedural applications, tailored to the specific anatomical and clinical challenges presented by the patient. These techniques range from extensive multi-vessel reconstructions for thoracoabdominal disease to more focused interventions for hostile infrarenal anatomy

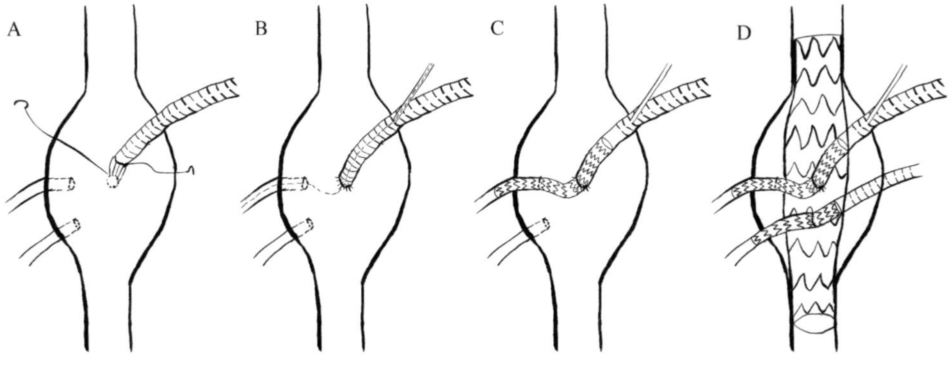

Figure 1.
Chunnel debranching technique – covered stent-channel configuration for visceral revascularization. (a) The inflow graft is anastomosed to the iliac artery and connected to the aneurysmal aortic wall. (b) A guidewire is advanced through the prosthetic graft into the target visceral branch. (c) A Viabahn stent graft is deployed across the aortic wall to create a covered conduit between the graft and the branch artery. (d) After completion of all channels, thoracic endovascular aortic repair (TEVAR) is performed to exclude the aneurysm sac.

and complex reoperative scenarios. The decision-making process, including the timing and specific configuration of the repair, is critical to achieving successful outcomes.

4.1 Thoracoabdominal aortic aneurysms

The treatment of TAAAs represents the most extensive and common application of the hybrid debranching principle.

4.1.1 Total abdominal debranching for Crawford Extent I–IV aneurysms

For TAAAs involving the visceral and renal arteries (Crawford Extents I–IV), total abdominal debranching followed by endovascular exclusion is the archetypal hybrid procedure [14]. This technique transforms a formidable single-stage open thoracoabdominal operation into two more manageable components: a major abdominal surgery and a standard thoracic endovascular aortic repair (TEVAR) [14, 20]. The open component involves creating retrograde bypasses from an aortoiliac inflow to the celiac, superior mesenteric, and both renal arteries, as previously described. Once perfusion to these vital organs is secured, the entire diseased thoracoabdominal aorta is rendered a passive conduit, which can be excluded with one or more overlapping tubular stent-grafts deployed from a healthy segment of the descending thoracic aorta down to the new infrarenal graft [6, 14]. This approach effectively avoids the morbidity associated with a thoracotomy, aortic cross-clamping above the diaphragm, and the potential need for extracorporeal circulatory support. A schematic illustration of the hybrid repair steps for an extent IV TAAA is presented in **Figure 2**.

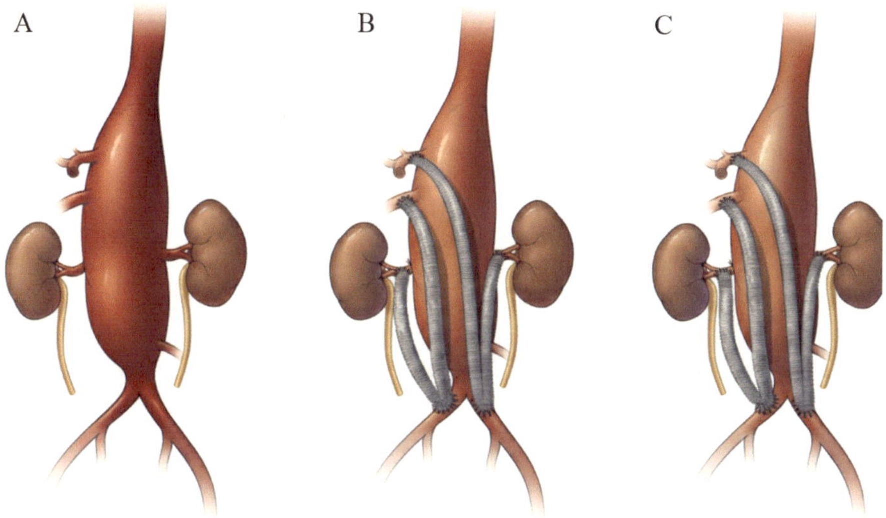

Figure 2.
Hybrid repair of an extent IV thoracoabdominal aortic aneurysm: stepwise schematic of debranching and TEVAR workflow. (a) Schematic representation of an Extent IV thoracoabdominal aortic aneurysm involving the visceral and renal branches. (b) Extra-anatomic revascularization of the celiac, superior mesenteric, and renal arteries with a bifurcated polyethylene terephthalate (Dacron) graft using bilateral iliac arteries as inflow. The native branches proximal to the bypass are ligated to prevent type II endoleaks. (c) Completion stage showing thoracic endovascular aortic repair (TEVAR) for aneurysm exclusion following debranching.

4.1.2 Staged versus single-stage repairs: A clinical dilemma

A key strategic consideration in hybrid TAAA repair is the timing of the open and endovascular procedures. A staged approach, where the visceral debranching is performed first and TEVAR is delayed for several days to weeks, is often advocated [6, 20]. The primary rationale for staging is to reduce the risk of SCI. The interval between procedures theoretically allows for the conditioning and recruitment of the spinal cord's collateral blood network before the segmental arteries are covered by the endograft. One study demonstrated a significantly higher incidence of SCI in patients who underwent TEVAR within three days of debranching compared to those with a longer interval [20]. However, this strategy carries the significant risk of interval aneurysm rupture, a fatal complication reported in up to 19% of patients in some series. One institution reported two in-hospital deaths from rupture while patients were awaiting the second stage of their repair.

Conversely, a single-stage procedure, where both the debranching and TEVAR are performed during the same anesthetic, eliminates the risk of interval rupture [20]. This approach is often preferred for patients with large (>60 mm), symptomatic, or contained ruptured aneurysms where the risk of a delay is deemed unacceptably high [19]. The decision between a staged versus single-stage repair remains a clinical judgment, balancing the risk of SCI against the risk of aneurysm rupture based on the patient's specific anatomy and clinical presentation.

4.2 Hostile infrarenal anatomy

Hybrid techniques are not limited to TAAAs and provide effective solutions for anatomically complex, purely infrarenal AAAs that are unsuitable for standard EVAR.

4.2.1 The "funnel technique" for wide aortic necks

A wide proximal aortic neck (>32 mm) is a common contraindication for standard EVAR because commercial abdominal endografts cannot achieve the necessary 10%–20% oversizing for a durable seal. The "Funnel Technique" (FT-EVAR) is an off-label hybrid solution that utilizes a large-diameter thoracic stent-graft as a proximal cuff to bridge this size mismatch. The procedure involves first deploying a standard bifurcated abdominal endograft distally, often with its flow divider seated on the aortic bifurcation. Subsequently, a thoracic stent-graft (available in diameters up to 46 mm) is deployed proximally, with its distal end telescoping inside the main body of the abdominal device to create a "funnel" shape [10]. This technique leverages off-the-shelf devices and is particularly useful in urgent cases or for high-risk patients with limited life expectancy. To enhance stability and mitigate the risk of late migration or type Ia endoleak, endoanchors can be used to fixate both the thoracic cuff and the abdominal endograft to the aortic wall, a modification known as the Cuff Plus Anchoring Funnel Technique (CAF-EVAR). A schematic representation of the FT-EVAR used for proximal sealing is shown in **Figure 3**.

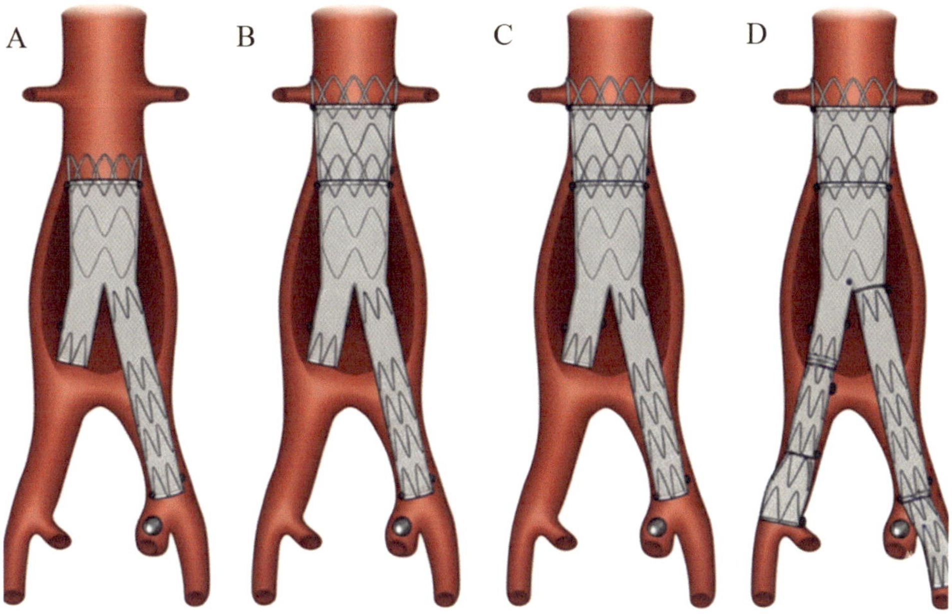

Figure 3.
Funnel technique (FT-EVAR): stepwise illustration of proximal sealing configuration. (a) After embolization of the left internal iliac artery, the main body of the bifurcated aortic stent graft is positioned within the aneurysm sac. (b) A straight thoracic endograft is advanced through the ipsilateral femoral access and deployed as a proximal extension of the bifurcated main body. (c) The left iliac limb extension is released into the left external iliac artery to complete distal sealing. (d) Sequential iliac extensions are added from the integral limb of the main body toward the right common iliac artery, forming a funnel-shaped proximal configuration that completes aneurysm exclusion.

4.2.2 Hybrid solutions for severe iliac artery occlusive disease and calcification

Hostile iliac anatomy, such as chronic total occlusion or severe circumferential calcification, poses a significant barrier to both open and endovascular repair. Hybrid techniques can overcome these challenges. For patients undergoing OSR with heavily calcified, non-clampable iliac arteries, a hybrid approach involves first gaining retrograde femoral access and deploying covered stent grafts into the common iliac arteries. The proximal ends of these stents are left within the aneurysm sac, and the limbs of the open surgical graft are then sewn directly to the stent grafts, creating a secure stent-to-graft anastomosis [8].

For patients with AAA and concomitant iliac artery occlusion who are candidates for EVAR, a hybrid approach involves first endovascularly recanalizing the occluded iliac segment from a contralateral or brachial approach. Once a channel is created, a standard bifurcated EVAR device can be deployed, with its contralateral limb passing through the newly opened segment and often reinforced with an additional covered stent to ensure long-term patency. In cases where the common femoral artery is also diseased, this can be combined with a surgical endarterectomy and patch angioplasty. This strategy allows for the successful implantation of a bifurcated endograft, avoiding the need for a less desirable aorto-uni-iliac (AUI) configuration with a femoro–femoral bypass [12].

4.3 Hybrid management of reoperative aortic scenarios

Patients with a history of prior aortic surgery represent a particularly high-risk group in whom hybrid techniques can minimize the morbidity of re-intervention.

4.3.1 TAAA repair after previous open AAA surgery

Patients with a prior open AAA repair may develop new or progressive aneurysmal disease in the thoracoabdominal segment. A conventional redo open repair in this setting is a formidable procedure due to extensive adhesions. A hybrid approach provides a safer alternative by utilizing the existing, well-incorporated abdominal graft as a stable inflow source for a new visceral debranching procedure. A quadrifurcated graft can be anastomosed directly to a limb or the body of the previous graft to revascularize the visceral vessels, followed by TEVAR to exclude the TAAA [20]. Studies have shown that this approach is safe and effective, with long-term survival and freedom from aortic events comparable to that of patients undergoing a primary hybrid repair.

4.3.2 Managing complications of prior repairs: Endoleaks, seromas, and pseudoaneurysms

Hybrid techniques serve a vital "bailout" or rescue function in managing late complications of both open and endovascular repairs. Late aneurysm rupture after EVAR can be caused by endoleaks, such as a type IIIb (fabric defect) endoleak, which may be difficult to diagnose or treat purely endovascularly. In such cases, a hybrid approach combining laparotomy with endovascular techniques can be life-saving. After establishing proximal control with an intra-aortic balloon, a limited laparotomy allows for sacotomy, evacuation of the hematoma, and direct identification of the endograft defect, which can then be relined with a new endograft from within [21].

Similarly, for rare complications of open repair, such as large, symptomatic perigraft seromas or para-anastomotic pseudoaneurysms (PAAs), a hybrid approach can reduce operative risk. A large seroma can be managed by endovascularly relining the original porous graft with a low-permeability covered stent graft to stop fluid ultrafiltration, combined with simultaneous open drainage of the fluid collection [22]. For PAAs, where surgical dissection for proximal control is hazardous due to severe adhesions, an endovascular occlusion balloon can be inserted from a remote access site to control inflow while the PAA is repaired surgically [16].

5. Special considerations and future directions

The application of hybrid techniques extends beyond elective, degenerative TAAAs to encompass a range of specialized and urgent clinical scenarios. The role of hybrid repair must also be viewed in the context of rapidly advancing total endovascular technologies, which shape its current and future position in the treatment algorithm for complex aortic disease.

5.1 Ruptured AAAs

5.1.1 The role of the hybrid emergency room and balloon occlusion

In the setting of a ruptured AAA (rAAA), time is critical, and hemodynamic instability is the primary driver of mortality [21, 23]. Hybrid strategies and facilities are uniquely suited to address this challenge. The "Hybrid Emergency Room" concept, an integrated suite equipped for simultaneous CT, interventional radiology, and open surgery, has been shown to drastically reduce the door-to-intervention time by eliminating patient transfers [7]. A key component of modern rAAA management, whether open, endovascular, or hybrid, is the rapid achievement of proximal aortic control. Percutaneous intra-aortic balloon occlusion (IABO), often performed under local anesthesia before the induction of general anesthesia, serves as a crucial bridge to definitive repair [23]. This technique provides temporary hemodynamic stability, allowing for a more controlled operative environment and facilitating either endovascular or open intervention. The "double-balloon technique," where balloons are used alternately from bilateral femoral access, has also been described to maintain continuous aortic occlusion while facilitating the deployment of endograft components.

5.1.2 Hybrid strategies for ruptures complicating a previous EVAR

Late rupture after a primary EVAR is a rare but life-threatening complication, often resulting from previously unidentified or undertreated endoleaks [21]. These cases are frequently complex due to the existing endograft and altered anatomy. Hybrid repair offers a versatile solution for such scenarios. In cases of rupture caused by a type III endoleak (component separation or fabric defect), a purely endovascular approach may be difficult [21, 24]. A hybrid strategy, combining a limited laparotomy with endovascular techniques, can be highly effective. After achieving proximal control with an aortic balloon, a sacotomy can be performed to evacuate the hematoma, directly identify the endograft defect, and control any back-bleeding from branch vessels like the inferior mesenteric artery (IMA) [21]. With the source of the leak identified and controlled, a new endograft can be deployed to reline the failing device, effectively sealing the defect from within. This approach is less invasive than a full endograft explantation and open conversion.

5.2 Patients with connective tissue disorders (e.g., Loeys–Dietz syndrome)

Patients with genetic aortopathies, such as Loeys–Dietz syndrome (LDS) or Marfan syndrome, present a unique challenge due to the inherent fragility of their aortic tissue. These patients often have extensive, multi-segmental aortic disease and frequently a history of multiple prior aortic surgeries. While open repair remains the gold standard for heritable aortopathies, the morbidity of re-operative open thoracoabdominal surgery is substantial [6]. A purely endovascular approach is often contraindicated because achieving a durable seal by anchoring an endograft to the weak, native aortic wall carries a high risk of new dissection or late treatment failure.

Hybrid repair provides a logical solution by creating durable, surgical graft-to-graft landing zones. By first performing an open repair on one segment (e.g., an infrarenal aortoiliac bypass) and subsequently deploying an endograft that lands proximally and distally within synthetic graft material, the reliance on diseased native tissue for sealing is eliminated, mitigating the primary failure mode of endovascular repair in this population.

5.3 Unique anatomical challenges: Post-renal transplant and poliomyelitis sequelae

Hybrid principles can be adapted to protect vital structures and overcome unusual anatomical barriers in special patient populations. In kidney transplant recipients with an AAA, aortic cross-clamping during OSR poses a significant risk of ischemic injury to the solitary renal allograft, which lacks collateral circulation. While EVAR can avoid clamping, it may not be anatomically feasible. In such cases, a hybrid technique involving a temporary, percutaneous brachiofemoral shunt can be used to provide continuous perfusion to the transplanted kidney and lower extremities during the open repair, serving as a safe and rapid method for renal allograft protection [25].

Severe musculoskeletal deformities, such as those resulting from poliomyelitis, can create profound anatomical challenges. A patient with severe scoliosis, a laterally deviated aneurysm, and an atrophic external iliac artery may be unsuitable for both a standard transperitoneal open approach and a standard EVAR. A hybrid repair, using a retroperitoneal approach to manage the deviated proximal aorta, combined with an endovascular stent graft (e.g., Viabahn) for the atrophic iliac limb, can facilitate a successful repair by minimizing the need for difficult contralateral dissection and anastomosis [9].

6. Conclusion

The management of complex abdominal and TAAAs represents a significant and evolving challenge in modern vascular surgery. While conventional open surgical repair remains a durable standard, and total endovascular techniques offer remarkable minimally invasive solutions, neither approach is universally applicable. The extensive literature reviewed in this chapter clearly establishes hybrid repair as an indispensable third pillar in the therapeutic armamentarium, occupying a crucial space for patients with prohibitive surgical risk and anatomies unsuitable for a purely endovascular solution.

The fundamental strength of the hybrid paradigm lies in its adaptability. By combining targeted open surgical revascularization with the reduced physiological burden of endovascular aneurysm exclusion, it provides effective solutions across a wide spectrum of clinical scenarios. This review has highlighted its primary role in treating extensive TAAAs through visceral debranching, its utility in managing hostile infrarenal necks via techniques like the "Funnel" procedure, and its capacity to overcome severe aortoiliac occlusive disease. Furthermore, the value of hybrid strategies in reoperative settings, both after previous open surgery and for managing late complications of endovascular repair, demonstrates its critical function as a problem-solving tool for some of the most challenging cases surgeons face.

Outcomes from hybrid procedures, as synthesized from the available literature, reflect the high-risk nature of the patient population for which they are reserved. While mortality and morbidity rates are not insignificant, they are often favorable when compared to the projected risks of extensive open repair in the same cohort. Complications such as SCI and renal failure remain pertinent concerns, driving the ongoing refinement of techniques like staged procedures and advanced intraoperative organ protection strategies. The data underscore that success is heavily dependent on meticulous patient selection, procedural planning, and institutional experience, reinforcing the need for these procedures to be performed in high-volume, specialized aortic centers.

In the contemporary era, the role of hybrid repair is defined by its complementary relationship with advancing fenestrated and branched endovascular technologies. While F/B-EVAR is increasingly the preferred approach for elective, anatomically suitable patients, hybrid repair retains its critical importance in urgent and emergent situations, for anatomies that preclude a total endovascular approach, and in healthcare systems where custom device manufacturing is not readily accessible. It is not a competing modality but a vital component of a comprehensive, patient-centered treatment algorithm. Future research, likely driven by large-scale international registries, is needed to further refine patient selection criteria, optimize long-term surveillance protocols, and solidify the position of hybrid techniques in the ever-evolving landscape of complex aortic surgery.

Author details

Ersin Ozer
Department of Cardiovascular Surgery, Ordu University Education and Research Hospital, Ordu, Türkiye

*Address all correspondence to: ersinozer@live.com

References

[1] Li DY, Busch A, Jin H, Chernogubova E, Pelisek J, Karlsson J, et al. H19 induces abdominal aortic aneurysm development and progression. Circulation. 2018;**138**:1551–1568

[2] Schmitz-Rixen T, Böckler D, Vogl TJ, Grundmann RT. Endovascular and open repair of abdominal aortic aneurysm. Deutsches Arzteblatt International. 2020;**117**(48):813–819. DOI: 10.3238/arztebl.2020.0813

[3] Anagnostakos J, Lal BK. Abdominal aortic aneurysms. Progress in Cardiovascular Diseases. 2021;**65**:34–43. DOI: 10.1016/j.pcad.2021.03.009

[4] Lu S, Wang R, Fu W, Si Y. Applications of extracellular vesicles in abdominal aortic aneurysm. Frontiers in Cardiovascular Medicine. 2022;**9**:927542. DOI: 10.3389/fcvm.2022.927542

[5] Blair R, Harkin D, Johnston D, Lim A, McFetridge L, Mitchell H. Open surgery for abdominal aortic aneurysm: 980 consecutive patient outcomes from a high-volume centre in the United Kingdom. Vascular and Endovascular Surgery. 2023;**57**(5):463–470. DOI: 10.1177/15385744221149585

[6] Naiem AA, Doonan RJ, Steinmetz OK. Hybrid repair of a thoraco-abdominal aortic aneurysm associated with Loeys-Dietz syndrome. European Journal of Vascular and Endovascular Surgery Vascular Forum. 2021;**51**:23–26. DOI: 10.1016/j.ejvsvf.2021.04.004

[7] Murai Y, Matsumoto S, Egawa T, Funabiki T, Shimogawara T. Hybrid emergency room management of a ruptured abdominal aortic aneurysm. Journal of Vascular Surgery Cases, Innovations and Techniques. 2021;**7**(1):21–25. DOI: 10.1016/j.jvscit.2020.12.006

[8] Krzyzaniak H, Misati G, Rockley M, Rommens K. Hybrid surgical technique for open abdominal aortic aneurysm repair in the setting of severe iliac artery calcification. Journal of Vascular Surgery Cases and Innovative Techniques. 2023;**9**(2):101141. DOI:10.1016/j.jvscit.2023.101141

[9] Yang SS. Hybrid repair of abdominal aortic aneurysm in a patient with poliomyelitis-related deformities. Journal of Vascular Surgery. 2018;**67**(3):945–948. DOI: 10.1016/j.jvs.2017.08.096

[10] Amico A, Russo D, Franciosi FB, Musio D, De Prisco R, Celoria G. Hybrid endografts in 'wide neck' abdominal aortic aneurysm in patients unfit for open surgery: The Funnel Technique – Case report and review of the literature. Vascular. 2021;**29**(4):509–515. DOI: 10.1177/1708538120962616

[11] Higashiura W. Endovascular treatment for thoracoabdominal aortic aneurysm and complex abdominal aortic aneurysm using fenestrated and branched grafts. Interventional Radiology. 2020;**5**(3):103–113. DOI: 10.22575/interventionalradiology.2020-0015

[12] Angiletta D, Wiesel P, Pisanello S, Patruno I, Pulli R. Endovascular and hybrid management of patients affected by abdominal aortic aneurysm and occlusion of the iliac arteries. Annals of Vascular Surgery. 2019;**56**:147–152. DOI: 10.1016/j.avsg.2018.08.093

[13] Ma X, Feng Y, Tardzenyuy MA, Qin B, Zhu Q, Akilu W, et al. Debranching abdominal aortic hybrid surgery for aortic diseases involving the visceral arteries. Frontiers in Cardiovascular Medicine. 2023;**10**:1219788. DOI: 10.3389/fcvm.2023.1219788

[14] Tanaka A, Oderich GS, Estrera AL. Total abdominal debranching hybrid thoracoabdominal aortic aneurysm repair versus chimneys and snorkels. Journal of Thoracic and Cardiovascular Surgery Techniques. 2021;**10**:28–33. DOI: 10.1016/j.xjtc.2021.08.002

[15] Elhelali A, Hynes N, Devane D, Sultan S, Kavanagh EP, Morris L, et al. Hybrid repair versus conventional open repair for thoracic aortic arch aneurysms. The Cochrane Database of Systematic Reviews. 2021;**6**:CD012923

[16] Moriuchi H, Shimabukuro N, Yamauchi A. Simultaneous repair of pseudo para-anastomotic aneurysm and abdominal aortic aneurysm with hybrid approach. Clinical Case Reports. 2025;**13**(10):e70999. DOI: 10.1002/ccr3.70999

[17] Wakasa S, Sato K, Ishigaki T, Watabe Y, Abe S. Chunnel debranching for hybrid repair of thoracoabdominal aortic aneurysm. General Thoracic and Cardiovascular Surgery. 2022;**70**(6):588–590. DOI: 10.1007/s11748-022-01805-7

[18] Kavanagh EP, Sultan S, Jordan F, Elhelali A, Devane D, Veerasingam D, et al. Hybrid repair versus conventional open repair for aortic arch dissection. The Cochrane Database of Systematic Reviews. 2021;**7**:CD012920

[19] Shuto T, Wada T, Miyamoto S, Kamei N, Hongo N, Mori H. Ten-year experience of the thoraco-abdominal aortic aneurysm treatment using a hybrid thoracic endovascular aortic repair. Interactive CardioVascular and Thoracic Surgery. 2018;**26**(6):951–956. DOI: 10.1093/icvts/ivy021

[20] Ueno K, Shuto T, Kawashima T, Wada T, Oji K, Dotsu T, et al. Hybrid thoracoabdominal aortic aneurysm repair after prior abdominal aortic aneurysm repair: Safety and outcomes. Interdisciplinary Cardiovascular and Thoracic Surgery. 2025;**40**:ivaf230. DOI: 10.1093/icvts/ivaf230

[21] Koizumi S, Hayashida N, Hasegawa H, Asano S. Successful hybrid management of a ruptured abdominal aortic aneurysm induced by type II and IIIB endoleaks after endovascular aortic repair. Journal of Vascular Surgery Cases, Innovations and Techniques. 2019;**5**(3):323–326. DOI: 10.1016/j.jvscit.2019.03.016

[22] Ono S, Obara H, Hagiwara K, Saida F, Oshiro K, Matsubara K, et al. A hybrid technique to manage a large perigraft seroma after an open abdominal aortic aneurysm repair: A case report. Annals of Vascular Surgery. 2019;**56**:352.e1–352.e4

[23] Nakayama H, Toma M, Kobayashi T, Ohno N, Okada T, Ueno G, Sato Y. Ruptured abdominal aortic aneurysm treated by double-balloon technique and endovascular strategy: Case series. Annals of Thoracic and Cardiovascular Surgery. 2019;**25**(4):211–214. DOI: 10.5761/atcs.cr.17-00189

[24] Nakano Y, Nishi S, Yamazaki Y, Yoshimoto A, Suematsu Y. Successful hybrid repair for ruptured abdominal aortic aneurysm caused by type IIIa endoleak resulting from a disconnected contralateral limb. Journal of Vascular Surgery Cases, Innovations and

Techniques. 2022;**8**(3):417–420. DOI: 10.1016/j.jvscit.2022.05.013

[25] Salimi J, Sadat SA, Barhaghtalab MJY, Rahimzadeh H. Hybrid percutaneous brachiofemoral shunt and open abdominal aortic aneurysm repair in a kidney transplant recipient. Case Reports in Vascular Medicine. 2021;**2021**:6655660. DOI: 10.1155/2021/6655660

Chapter 7

Aortoiliac Disease: Current Management

Pedro Adolfo Mera Almonte

Abstract

The chapter offers up-to-date and timely information, covering everything from clinical diagnosis, noninvasive vascular laboratory testing, and imaging, to conservative medical management (tobacco cessation, lifestyle changes, diet, blood pressure control, glycemic control), endovascular management, and the various open surgical techniques. Regarding endovascular management or open surgery, emphasis will be placed on the best indications according to the patient's perioperative risk, the anatomical distribution of stenosis or occlusions in the aortoiliac segment based on current classification systems, and the best-reported results. Follow-up recommendations, detection of restenosis or occlusion as appropriate, and management recommendations for these situations will be included. Current statistical data and profiles of people at risk for aortoiliac disease will also be included.

Keywords: aortoiliac disease, CERAB technique, aortoiliac bypass, aortobifemoral bypass, axillary–femoral bypass

1. Introduction

The treatment of aortoiliac disease has been based, for the most part, on endovascular strategies, regardless of the Transatlantic Intersociety Consensus (TASC) classification grade. Traditionally, open surgery is performed in patients with high-grade calcification of the disease or when endovascular procedures fail. While open surgery offers adequate long-term patency, it can also be associated with significant perioperative morbidity. TASC C and D lesions, when treated endovascularly, have been reported to result in patency rates comparable to traditional open surgery [1]. In this sense, there has been a paradigm shift in the recommendations made by different societies, which now recommend endovascular therapy as the first-line treatment and primary approach for aortoiliac disease, whether diffuse or focal. However, endovascular therapy has both advantages and disadvantages. This article aims to present the relevant recommendations for the management of aortoiliac disease from a current perspective, as well as the therapeutic challenges posed by each method.

2. Aortoiliac disease

Aortoiliac artery disease (AIAD), which causes occlusion or narrowing of this segment, is mostly caused by cholesterol plaques or atherosclerosis extending from the infrarenal abdominal aorta to the iliac artery. As with other peripheral arterial diseases (PADs), AIAD affects blood flow to the organs contained in the pelvis and lower extremities, either by narrowing the lumen, total occlusion, or plaque embolization. Risk factors include homocysteinemia, tobacco use, dyslipidemia or hypercholesterolemia, diabetes mellitus, and systemic arterial hypertension. Non-modifiable risk factors include age, race, sex, and family history. Takayasu's artery disease, although rare, is a significant risk factor [2].

As the population ages steadily due to increasing life expectancy, there has also been an increasing incidence of PAD. In countries such as the United States, prevalence estimates indicate that between 7 and 12 million people are affected, with estimates of 200 million worldwide. However, these data depend on how the disease is defined; including only symptomatic patients leads to an underestimation when reporting the disease. The rate of PAD increases with age, with a higher prevalence in those over 70 years of age. On the contrary, it is estimated that severe PAD with chronic limb-threatening ischemia (CLTI) affects 1.3% of cases and can lead to amputation [1].

Patients often present with cramping or claudication, which are usually associated with physical activity and relieved with rest. A complete physical examination and detailed clinical history are essential to define the degree of severity and differentiate it from other conditions. Pain located more proximally usually indicates severe stenosis or proximal occlusion. The triad of proximal claudication, absent femoral pulses, and sexual dysfunction, described by Leriche and Morel, is the most common clinical manifestation of aortoiliac occlusive disease (AIOD). The presentation of the disease can vary from asymptomatic to clinical signs and symptoms with severe limb-threatening ischemia. Patients may present to the physician's office or emergency department with symptoms and signs of severe stenosis or complete obstruction, or due to an acute limb-threatening embolic event. The clinical features and diagnostic criteria for CLTI include ischemic rest pain, gangrene, or ulceration in the lower extremities that persist for more than two weeks in patients with PAD. The possibility of an acute episode should also be assessed.

The therapeutic management of AIOD regularly results in significant symptom improvement, even in the presence of distal arterial disease. Invasive surgical procedures to treat this anatomical segment have been replaced by endovascular techniques (primary stenting, balloon angioplasty with selective stenting, etc.).

2.1 Diagnostic

Diagnostic evaluation is included in the concept of PAD. When aortoiliac disease is suspected, an approach that includes history (gluteal claudication, impotence in men, and absent femoral pulses in patients with defined risk factors), physical examination, ankle–brachial index (ABI), finger–brachial index, pulse volume recording (PVR), as well as arterial Doppler and invasive imaging (angiography/computed tomography [CT] angiography) is essential (see **Figure 1**).

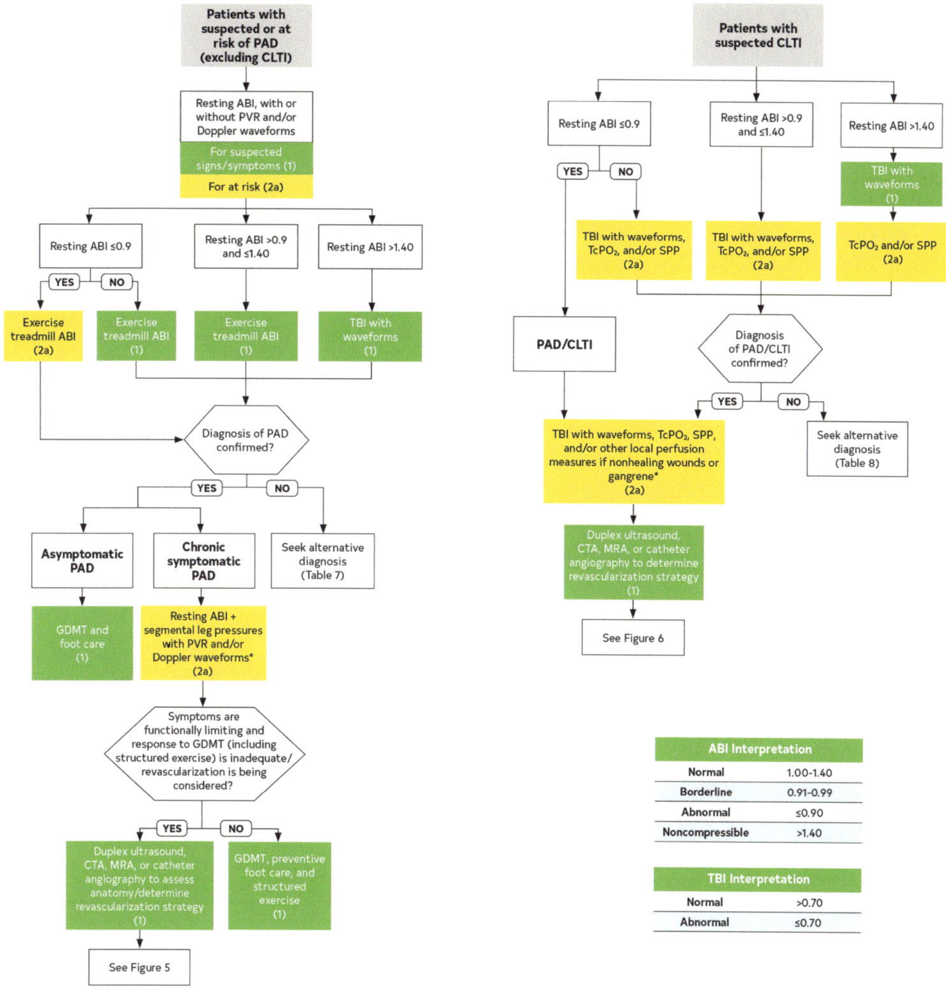

Figure 1.
Algorithm for diagnostic testing for PAD. Gornik et al. [3].

The proper use of these diagnostic methods allows us to appropriately utilize resources such as revascularization in patients who may require treatment. Furthermore, it helps avoid unnecessary testing in patients for whom further delineation of the arterial anatomy will not affect treatment plans [3]. Arterial imaging is reserved for instances when revascularization is being considered or if clinical features of PAD are present but the ABI and physiologic studies are inconclusive. Imaging methods include arterial duplex, CT angiography, angiography, and magnetic resonance (MR) angiography; contrast-enhanced images demonstrate anatomical details, the distribution and complexity of PAD, and aortoiliac disease. Catheter angiography, like the aforementioned methods, is generally limited to the most severe presentations of PAD and aortoiliac disease, where revascularization is being considered and the benefits outweigh the risks of potential complications associated with contrast and radiation [3].

2.2 Clinical classification

Classification systems for PAD, both clinical and anatomical and radiological, provide clinicians with accepted and periodically updated criteria for the evaluation, treatment, management, and follow-up of patients, and are a valuable tool for research and subsequent recommendations, as they facilitate the objective comparison of different treatment strategies.

Rutherford classifies PAD into acute and chronic limb ischemia, considering that each presentation will require different therapeutic strategies, approaches, and algorithms. The La Fontaine classification assigns a degree of severity based solely on clinical symptoms, without other diagnostic tests [4, 5] (see **Figures 2** and **3**).

Ischemia represents one of the three factors that put a limb at risk for amputation. The SVS devised a classification system according to the severity of each of these

Grade	Category	Clinical description	Objective criteria
0	0	Asymptomatic-no hemodynamically significant occlusive disease	Normal treadmill or reactive hyperemia test
	1	Mild claudication	Completes treadmill exercise; AP after exercise > 50 mmHg but at least 20 mmHg lower than resting value
I	2	Moderate claudication	Between categories 1 and 3
	3	Severe claudication	Cannot complete standard treadmill exercise, and AP after exercise < 50 mm Hg
II	4	Ischemic rest pain	Resting AP < 40 mmHg, flat or barely pulsatile ankle or metatarsal PVR; TP < 30 mm Hg
III	5	Minor tissue loss non-healing ulcer, focal gangrene with diffuse pedal ischemia	Resting AP < 60 mm Hg, ankle or metatarsal PVR flat or barely pulsatile; TP < 40 mm Hg
	6	Major tissue loss-extending above TM level, functional foot no longer salvageable	Same as category 5

AP: ankle pressure; PVR: pulse volume recording; TM: transmetatarsal; TP: toe pressure.

Figure 2.
Rutherford classification for chronic limb ischemia. Desai et al. [4].

Increasing severity		Symptom complex	Rutherford Classification	Fontaine Classification
		Asymptomatic	Stage 0	Stage I
	Intermittent claudication	Mild Claudication	Stage 1	Stage II A (symptomatic upon > 200m walking
		Moderate claudication	Stage 2	Stage II B (symptomatic < 200m walking)
		Severe claudication	Stage 3	
	Critical limb ischemia	Rest pain	Stage 4	Stage III
		Ischemia ulceration	Stage 5	Stage IV
		Severe ulceration or gangrene	Stage 6	

Figure 3.
The Fontaine classification system assigns severity based entirely on clinical symptoms without other diagnostic tests. Dave et al. [5].

factors: wound, ischemia, and infection (WIfI) of the foot. The classification system is based on severity, where 0 represents none, 1 represents mild, 2 represents moderate, and 3 represents severe. This classification is a synthesis of several previously published classification schemes, merging systems focused on diabetic foot ulcers and pure ischemia models [6] (see **Figure 4**).

a, Estimate risk of amputation at 1 year for each combination

	Ischemia – 0				Ischemia – 1				Ischemia – 2				Ischemia – 3			
W-0	VL	VL	L	M	VL	L	M	H	L	L	M	H	L	M	M	H
W-1	VL	VL	L	M	VL	L	M	H	L	M	H	H	M	M	H	H
W-2	L	L	M	H	M	M	H	H	M	H	H	H	H	H	H	H
W-3	M	M	H	H	H	H	H	H	H	H	H	H	H	H	H	H
	fI-0	fI-1	fI-2	fI-3	fI-0	fI-1	fI-2	fI-3	fI-0	fI-1	fI-2	fI-3	fI-0	fI-1	fI-2	fI-3

b, Estimate likelihood of benefit of/requirement for revascularization (assuming infection can be controlled first)

	Ischemia – 0				Ischemia – 1				Ischemia – 2				Ischemia – 3			
W-0	VL	VL	VL	VL	VL	L	L	M	L	L	M	M	M	H	H	H
W-1	VL	VL	VL	VL	L	M	M	M	M	H	H	H	H	H	H	H
W-2	VL	VL	VL	VL	M	M	H	H	H	H	H	H	H	H	H	H
W-3	VL	VL	VL	VL	M	M	M	H	H	H	H	H	H	H	H	H
	f-0	fI-1	fI-2	fI-3	fI-0	fI-1	fI-2	fI-3	fI-0	fI-1	fI-2	fI-3	fI-0	fI-1	fI-2	fI-3

fI, foot Infection; I, Ischemia; W, Wound.

Premises:

1. Increase in wound class increases risk of amputation (based on PEDIS, UT, and other wound classification systems)
2. PAD and infection are synergistic (Eurodiale); infected wound + PAD increases likelihood revascularization will be needed to heal wound
3. Infection 3 category (systemic/metabolic instability): moderate to high-risk of amputation regardless of other factors (validated IDSA guidelines)

Four classes: for each box, group combination into one of these four classes

Very low = VL = clinical stage 1
Low = L = clinical stage 2
Moderate = M = clinical stage 3
High = H = clinical stage 4
Clinical stage 5 would signify an unsalvageable foot

Figure 4.
SVS WIfI classification system. Mills et al. [6].

2.3 Anatomic classification

2.3.1 TASC document II (TASC II)

The TASC II plays a fundamental and important role in treatment management for PAD and, in this case, aortoiliac disease.

Its use has had a significant impact on therapeutic decision-making and patient outcomes. Depending on the extent of the disease, the use of endovascular therapy or open surgery has been recommended [7, 8]. However, with advances in endovascular surgery, innovative devices, and improved outcomes over time, the complexity and distribution of aortoiliac disease are no longer limiting factors.

Ogunsanya et al. [9] have described a new classification system for AIOD. This classification includes the common femoral segments, as they serve as the distal access. Furthermore, the extent of the disease is important; this is essential for the planning and execution of procedures, whether open or endovascular. In this proposed classification, aortoiliac and femoral disease are classified according to severity. This helps create a descriptive map of the affected segments and defines the segments that require treatment, allowing for the creation of a surgical plan rather than recommending a specific strategy. The objective is solely to identify the lesion without emphasizing hemodynamic changes. A 50% stenosis in cross-sections was arbitrarily chosen to determine the need for treatment in a specific arterial segment.

3. Aortic–iliac disease: Treatment

3.1 Medical therapy

Medical treatment of PAD caused by aortoiliac disease is based on three fundamental pillars.

First, risk factors must be identified and managed intensively. Smoking and diabetes are the most important; therefore, it is imperative that the patient completely and permanently quit smoking. Blood glucose levels must be carefully regulated; the goal is to reduce glycated hemoglobin (HbA1c) to a level below 7% [10]. The goal for the management and control of high blood pressure is a level below 140/90 mmHg. LDL cholesterol should be reduced to less than 100 mg/dL; this is generally achieved with the use of statins (hepatic 3-methylglutaryl coenzyme A (HMG-CoA) reductase inhibitors) along with risk factor modification. These patients should receive lifelong antiplatelet agents to reduce the risk of myocardial infarction, stroke, and death from cardiovascular causes.

Prospective randomized clinical trials support and confirm the efficacy of walking for the management of claudication [11, 12]. Improvements of up to 180%–340% in the distance walked have been demonstrated. Supervised walking [13] has been shown to have better results than unsupervised exercise. Supervised walking reduces claudication pain due to improved efficiency of muscle enzymes involved in oxygen extraction and utilization.

There are two pharmacological agents currently approved by the US Food and Drug Administration (FDA), pentoxifylline and cilostazol; both can significantly improve claudication symptoms. Pentoxifylline, a methylxanthine derivative, acts as a hemorrheological agent, decreasing blood viscosity. However, it is effective in only 30%–40% of patients. When effective, it causes only a modest improvement in walking distance.

Cilostazol has been shown to be more effective and to offer better outcomes than pentoxifylline. This drug is generally well-tolerated; however, adverse effects may occur, including headache and diarrhea. It is contraindicated in patients with congestive heart failure.

3.2 Endovascular, open surgery, and hybrid procedure

In 1985, Julio Palmaz developed the first intraluminal stent, which represented a drastic change in endovascular treatment and its outcomes. However, despite all the advances in endovascular therapy, bypass grafting in its different forms remained the treatment of choice; this was due to its good long-term patency (confidence interval [CI]: 85%–92%, CI: 78%–83%) [14]. Nevertheless, perioperative morbidity and mortality rates are considerable.

In recent decades, continued evolution and advances in the development of materials and components, as well as techniques, have led to endovascular techniques for the treatment of aortoiliac disease increasingly replacing open surgery, given that minimally invasive methods offer lower mortality and morbidity.

In 2007, the TASC II guidelines were published [8], recommending endovascular treatment for type A and B lesions and open surgery for type C and D lesions (see **Figure 5**). TASC II recommends endovascular therapy for type C lesions, which have a low chance of cure after surgical revascularization. For TASC-II D lesions, which are very complex and extensive, conventional surgery has been the standard of care. However, in recent years, the guidelines have expanded the indications for endovascular therapy, especially in patients with high perioperative risk [15].

Jongkind et al. published a meta-analysis of endovascular therapy for extensive TASC-II D lesions (AIOD TASC C and D), which included 19 nonrandomized cohort studies with a total of 1,711 patients. Although primary patency at four and five years in the endovascular group was statistically inferior to that of open surgery (60%–86%), secondary patency results were similar (80%–98%), and, when necessary, most reoperations were performed endovascularly. For this meta-analysis, the endovascular approach was retrospectively compared with open surgery, and a significantly shorter hospital stay and perioperative morbidity were observed in the endovascular therapy group. The endovascular group showed significantly lower primary patency rates at three and four years (69% vs. 93%, $p = 0.013$ and 74% vs. 93%, $p = 0.002$); however, secondary patency was comparable between the two techniques (89% vs. 100%, $p > 0.05$ and 95% vs. 97%, $p = 0.3$) [16, 17].

The retrospective study by M. Freyermuth et al. [15], conducted at a tertiary center, included patients who were treated for lesions classified as symptomatic TASC-II D, requiring treatment of the aortoiliac bifurcation, with therapeutic approaches classified as purely percutaneous or hybrid surgery, over a 10-year period. The primary objective was to describe the long-term patency outcomes. Primary patency was 71.6%, assisted primary patency was 82.1%, and secondary

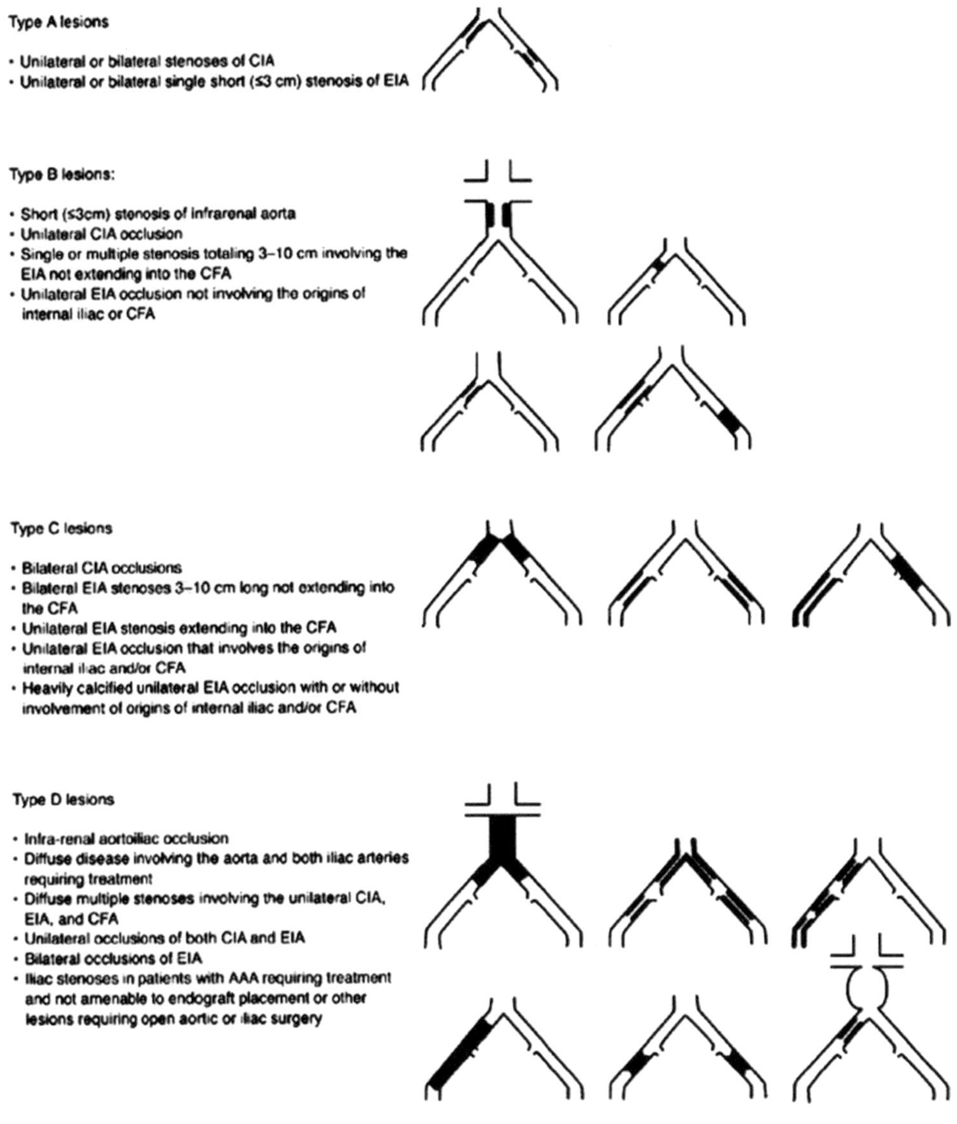

Figure 5.
The TASC II Classification of aortoiliac lesions.

patency was 96.3% over a period of five years. Regarding primary patency, a significant difference was found favoring the coated stent group at 36 months ($p < 0.01$) and at 60 months ($p = 0.037$). The overall complication rate was 11% [15].

The report by Mariana Basílio-Martins et al. [18], which compared the outcomes of open surgery and the endovascular approach for TASC-II D aortoiliac reconstruction in a total of 89 patients (open repair: 61, endovascular repair: 28) over a seven-year period, revealed that the technical success rate for the open approach was 100% versus 73.7% for the endovascular technique. There were no differences between the two groups in terms of complications, such as major adverse cardiovascular events (MACE) and major adverse limb events (MALE).

A review of clinical outcomes was conducted comparing hybrid surgery and endovascular therapy for the treatment of TASC-II D aortoiliac occlusion [19]. Patients underwent initial surgical treatment between March 2018 and March 2021. A perioperative mortality rate of 1.44% was observed in a total of 132 patients. One hundred twenty patients were treated with endovascular therapy (110 underwent stenting and 10 required thrombolysis prior to stenting), ten were treated with a hybrid procedure, and two with open surgery. At the end of follow-up, the hybrid group showed a patency rate of 100%, while the endovascular group had a patency rate of 89.17%. At the endline, the primary patency was 94.12% at 6 months, 92.44% at 12 months, and 89.08% at 24 months for the endovascular group, while for the hybrid group, it remained at 100%, with no significant differences between the two groups.

3.3 Recommendations for choosing the approach

Both open and endovascular techniques are effective and safe methods for the management of aortoiliac disease, including complex aortoiliac disease. Open repair is estimated to have a higher technical success rate; however, there are no significant differences in MACE or MALE between the two approaches [18].

The Transatlantic Trial for the Management of PAD (TASC II) has suggested that patients with TASC C and D aortoiliac disease receive surgical treatment, while TASC A and B patients should be managed with endovascular treatment [8]. Patients with TASC C and D often have multiple comorbidities and are unsuitable for open surgery, and an endovascular approach is increasingly preferred regardless of the type of injury. The foregoing supports the consideration of an endovascular approach for TASC-II D lesions in patients with severe comorbidities and at high surgical risk. However, it is suggested that this approach should be performed in experienced centers.

Even today, there is no defined consensus on the best strategy for the TASC-II C and D classifications. However, it is understood that the therapeutic strategy must be individualized according to the patient's physiological substrate, comorbidities, and risk factors, as well as age and life expectancy, to determine the most effective, safe, and long-lasting method.

3.4 Surgical therapy

3.4.1 Thromboendarterectomy

Thromboendarterectomy was the first surgical procedure for the management of aortoiliac disease. It is a relatively simple procedure, given that there is a demarcated plane between the medial layer and the obstructive plaque. By accessing the correct anatomical plane, the plaque, the internal elastic lamina, and the arterial intima are removed in a single piece. It is no longer used as frequently today. It is best utilized in combination as part of an aortoiliac or aortobifemoral bypass. It was developed by Dos Santos, and later the semi-closed technique was introduced, followed by eversion endarterectomy. The improved results in the long-term patency of aortofemoral bypass have led most surgeons to abandon this technique [19].

3.4.2 Aortic–bifemoral bypass

Aortoiliac bypass has been the most widely used open surgical technique. With increasing experience using the common femoral artery as an outflow route, primary patency has been achieved with optimal long-term results. Access can be transabdominal or retroperitoneal; the latter is preferred by some based on the theoretical benefit of fewer pulmonary complications and faster resolution of postoperative ileus. It has been the most widely used open surgical technique. After gaining more experience, it became clear that using the common femoral arteries as an outflow route offered better long-term patency results. Access can be transabdominal or retroperitoneal; the latter is preferred by some based on the theoretical benefit of fewer pulmonary complications and faster resolution of postoperative ileus. As mentioned above, endovascular revascularization has replaced aortobifemoral bypass as the first line of treatment. However, in patients for whom endovascular methods are unsuitable or unsuccessful, aortobifemoral bypass remains an important strategy and could be considered the standard due to its long-term patency [20].

Common indications include severe symptomatic atherosclerosis of the iliac artery or abdominal aorta, acute occlusion of the aorta or iliac arteries, persistent or recurrent claudication despite optimal medical therapy, leg ischemia or non-healing ulcers, critical limb ischemia manifesting as pain at rest or severe symptoms of claudication, and impotence [21]. In most cases, patency is high, with a five-year primary patency rate of 64% to 95% [22].

For this procedure, the patient is placed supine. The arms are abducted at 90 degrees. The skin is prepared from the nipples to the knees. Each common, deep, and superficial femoral artery is dissected bilaterally through inguinal incisions. Care must be taken to ensure that the arterial segments are healthy for adequate cross-clamping. Aortic exposure is achieved through a transperitoneal or retroperitoneal approach. The aorta is dissected below the renal arteries. If necessary, the renal vein can be mobilized by ligating its tributaries. Aortic exposure is achieved up to the point of emergence of the inferior mesenteric artery. Tunnels are made in the retroperitoneum, posterior to the ureters, extending to the inguinal incisions. Heparin (70–100 units/kg) is administered with a target transient time of action (TTA) of 250–300 seconds, and then the aorta is clamped infrarenally and in the already exposed distal portion. The aorta is dissected and divided into a segment generally proximal to the inferior mesenteric artery. The distal aorta is ligated. The bifurcated graft is anastomosed to the proximal aorta, usually end-to-side, with a 3–0 or 4–0 Prolene suture in running stitches. The graft branches are washed with heparinized saline solution, clamped, and inserted through the tunnels to the inguinal incisions. Vascular controls are placed for the femoral arteries, and an arteriotomy is performed up to the level of the deep femoral artery. If necessary, an endarterectomy and femoral artery graft are performed. The graft is anastomosed continuously end-to-side with a 4–0 or 5–0 Prolene suture. Before completing the anastomosis, retrograde and antegrade blood flow and irrigation are confirmed. Blood flow is released as follows: first to the common femoral artery, then to the deep femoral artery, and finally to the superficial femoral artery. Before unclamping, the anesthesiologist should be notified due to possible hypotension caused by reperfusion. The retroperitoneum should be closed routinely to prevent graft penetration into the gastrointestinal tract. If a cuff closure of the retroperitoneum is not possible, an omental flap should be created (see **Figure 6**) [22–25].

Significant complications include myocardial infarction, renal dysfunction, and significant respiratory disturbances. Late complications include hernias, graft thrombosis, graft pseudoaneurysms, graft infections, and aortoenteric fistulas. Acute myocardial infarction is the most common cause of death after aortofemoral bypass. The mortality rate associated with this surgical procedure is 1% to 2.5%. Renal failure occurs due to prolonged ischemia following aortic cross-clamping, embolization secondary to cross-clamping, hypoperfusion, hypovolemia, or intrinsic renal artery disease. Thrombosis may occur in up to 30% of patients.

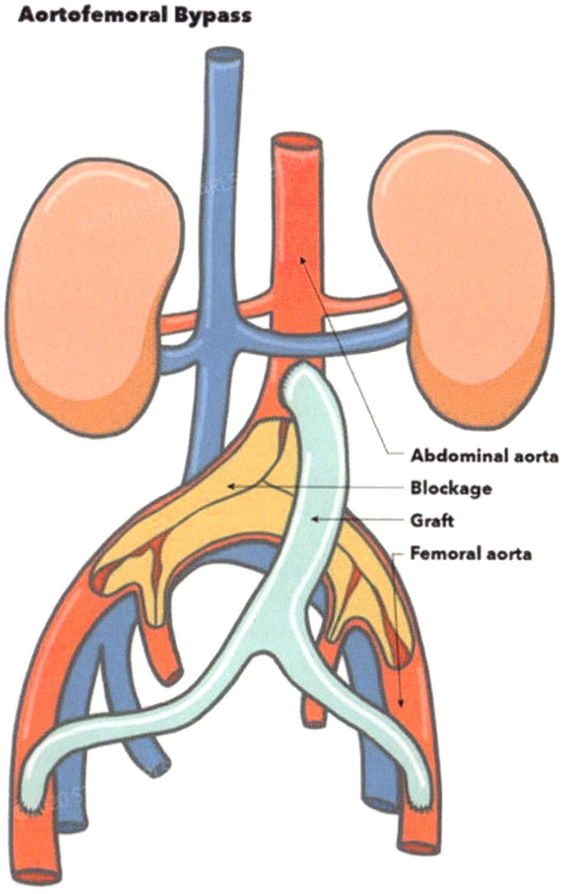

Figure 6.
Aortic-bifemoral by-pass. Dellehunt et al. [22].

Pseudoaneurysm, as a late complication, occurs in 1% to 5% of cases. Relatively rare, aortoenteric fistula tends to be devastating and fatal. The mortality rate is at least 30% in most cases. Management requires urgent exploratory laparotomy with graft explantation, debridement of infected tissue, bowel repair/resection, and extraanatomical bypass or placement of a new graft [22].

3.4.3 Axillofemoral bypass

Conditions at higher risk for complications after aortofemoral bypass surgery include retroperitoneal fibrosis, significant heart disease, recent myocardial infarction, multiple prior abdominal surgeries, horseshoe kidney, or recent stroke. End-stage renal disease constitutes a high-risk surgical group. Therefore, a high-risk condition that makes general anesthesia prohibitive is an absolute contraindication for aortofemoral bypass. These patients, whose anatomy is unfavorable for an endovascular procedure, are candidates for axillofemoral bypass as a surgical alternative.

The reported patency rate for bilateral axillofemoral bypasses has been 75% at two years, compared to 50% at two years for unilateral grafts. The five-year patency rate for axillobifemoral grafts varies between 30% and 85% [8]. While these figures are not comparable with the results of conventional aortobifemoral bypasses, they are performed in high-risk patients with no other therapeutic options [26].

A transverse incision is made 3 cm below the clavicle, exposing the pectoral muscle and dividing its fibers. The fat pad is dissected, and the vein, artery, and brachial plexus are exposed and inspected. The vein must be mobilized inferiorly to access the artery. A 3–4 cm segment of the artery is isolated, and branches are monitored at this level. Depending on the need, unilateral or bilateral exposure of the femoral arteries is performed in a routine and controlled manner. Longitudinal inguinal incisions are recommended. If the femoral sheath is accessed, the femoral arteries are dissected and controlled. The circumflex branches must be preserved. Subcutaneous tunneling is performed before systemic heparinization. The tunnel is created with a graft tunneling device in the midaxillary line, lateral to the breast and superior to the abdominal fascia, from the subclavian incision to the inguinal incision. When necessary, a femoral–femoral bridge is created superior to the pubic bone. The grafts are passed, ensuring there are no kinks. Systemic heparin is administered prior to vascular control and the anastomosis. The axillary anastomosis is initially performed. Adequate vascular control is achieved with angled vascular clamps. This is followed by longitudinal arteriotomy and cobra head grafting. An end-to-side anastomosis is constructed with a running stitch suture. The graft entry and exit of the distal axillary artery should be assessed. When a bifemoral configuration is required, the distal femorofemoral anastomosis (prosthesis–prosthesis) is first created and configured so that the distal axillary graft is ipsilateral to the femorofemoral anastomosis. Several brands offer prefabricated prostheses for this purpose. Vascular control is performed, and a longitudinal arteriotomy is created in the common femoral artery. A suitable end-to-side anastomosis is created (prosthesis–artery). If a significant artery is detected, the anastomosis is configured to include the deep femoral artery. If necessary, an endarterectomy should be performed on the recipient vessel (see **Figures** 7 and **8**) [26].

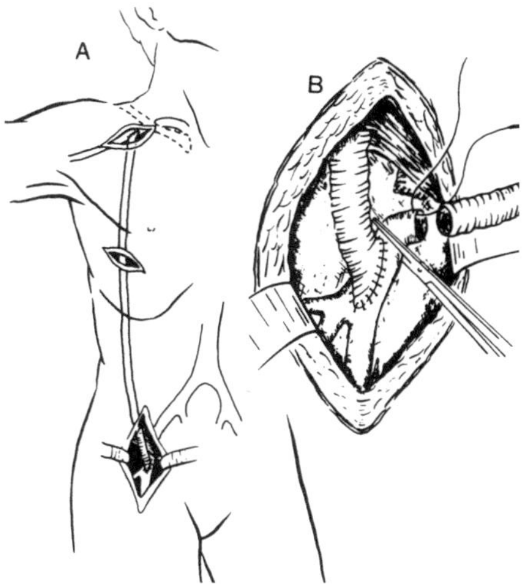

Figure 7.
Location of the proximal anastomosis for an axillofemoral graft. The segment of the artery used should be that extending from the clavicle to the pectoralis minor tendon.

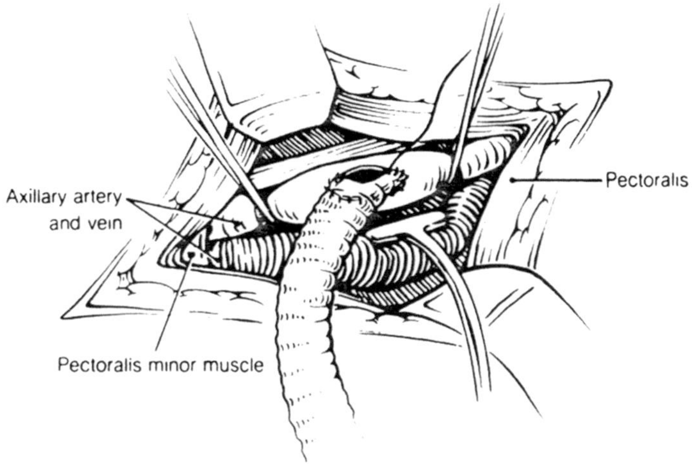

Figure 8.
Placement of the proximal femorofemoral graft anastomosis. Optimally, it should be as shown. The common femoral artery is divided at the inguinal ligament, and the distal end is used for the proximal graft anastomosis. Development of femoro–femoral and axillo–femoral bypass procedures Blaisdell, F. William. Journal of Vascular Surgery, Vol. 532, 540–544 *[26].*

3.4.4 Endovascular treatment

Treatment for the aortoiliac segment has historically been largely guided by the TASC II guidelines: endovascular treatment with stenting is recommended for less advanced disease, specifically TASC II A and B lesions, while surgery is recommended for more advanced lesions, TASC II C and D [8]. However, because open surgery for advanced lesions represents a high probability of complications, and considering the advancement of endovascular techniques and the development of better experiences, primary endovascular management with stenting has been recommended [27].

At a two-year follow-up, in a retrospective report after covered endovascular reconstruction of aortic bifurcation (CERAB) [28], patients classified as TASC II B, C, and D had a 100% technical success rate. During continued follow-up at 36 months, the primary patency, assisted primary patency, and secondary patency rates were 85%, 90%, and 92.5%, respectively. In another study, Dong, X. et al. reported the 10-year experience of endovascular treatment of AIOD with TASC II C and D lesions. Technical success was achieved in 96.2%. Significant improvement was observed in the ABI (preoperative 0.33 ± 0.14 vs. 1.0 ± 0.09). Primary patency rates were 100%, 95.7%, and 91.3% at one, three, and five years, respectively, with secondary patency rates of 100%. No deaths or serious complications related to the procedure were reported [29]. In the report on the long-term outcomes of endovascular reconstruction for AIOD, a retrospective cohort study presented by Gao Z. et al. [29], which evaluated the patency rate at 12, 36, and 60 months, technical success was reported in 98.7% of cases, with complications in 4.5%. Primary patency was 96.5%, 88.3%, and 80.4% at 12, 36, and 60 months, respectively, with secondary patency rates of 99%, 96.4%, and 88%, respectively. No significant differences were observed between A/B and C/D lesions for primary patency, secondary patency, or absence of TLR [30].

Therefore, endovascular reconstruction of the aortoiliac segment is safe and effective, with adequate patency rates and low surgical risk. It should be considered as a first-line treatment for TASC II A–D aortoiliac disease, always taking into account the patient profile [27–30]. A primary endovascular approach should be considered for all patients with aortoiliac disease. Various strategies and stent types are available for this approach. Currently, there is no consensus on which strategy and stent type are most appropriate. However, for severe disease involving the common iliac artery, the scientific literature supports the direct implantation of a balloon-expandable stent. A recent innovation in this field is the polytetrafluoroethylene (PTFE)-coated stent, which could further improve the primary patency of iliac stenting [31]. The results of the COBEST trial, a prospective, randomized, controlled clinical study, measured the outcomes of balloon-expandable stents, both covered and uncovered. Covered stents were more likely to remain free of restenosis at 18 months. It was also observed that the lesions that benefited most from the covered stent were TASC C and D [32].

3.4.4.1 Covered endovascular reconstruction of aortic bifurcation

CERAB is a safe and effective therapy for the management of these injuries. It offers a short hospital stay, a low perioperative morbidity rate, and zero mortality. It has also achieved satisfactory results in terms of primary patency [32]. Primary patency at 12, 24, and 36 months was reported to be 94.4%, 84.4%, and 83.8%, respectively. The reported complication rate was 11.7% [33].

The CERAB technique was introduced in 2013 with the goal of optimizing the outcomes of kissing stents, which have traditionally been the preferred endovascular technique. CERAB aims to improve arterial geometry and flow

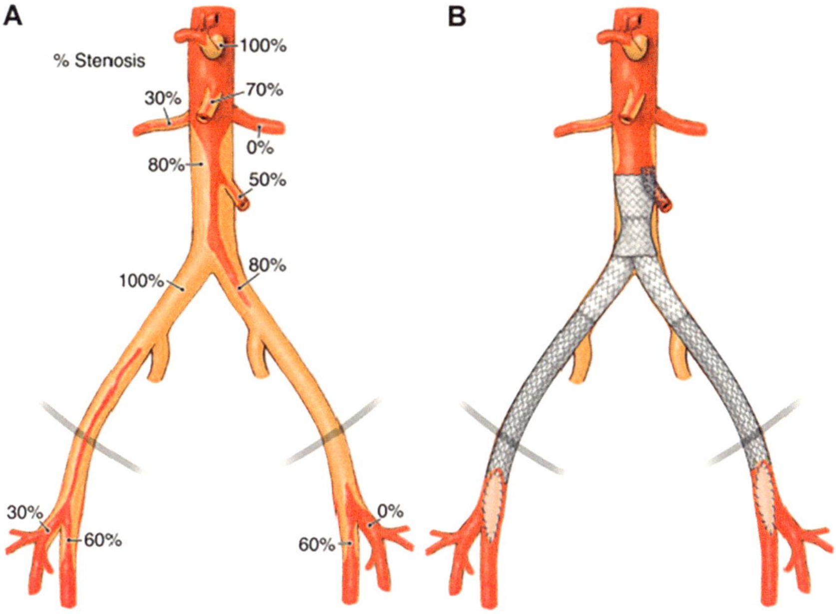

Figure 9.
Illustration of (a) preoperative computed tomography angiogram demonstrating high-grade infrarenal aortic stenosis and concomitant mesenteric stenosis. (b) Covered endovascular reconstruction of the aortic bifurcation with inferior mesenteric artery (IMA) chimney (CERAB) and bilateral femoral artery endarterectomy.

patterns. In CERAB, aortic reconstruction is performed with the implantation of three tightly connected, balloon-expandable covered stents, with adequate apposition to the wall, thus maintaining the geometric mismatch (see **Figures 9** and **10**) [34].

3.4.4.2 Kissing stent technique

The kissing stent technique has provided good results in patients with obstructive aortoiliac disease, without presenting a greater increase in immediate and intermediate-term complications, therefore representing an effective solution for aortoiliac disease [35]. This technique achieved technical success in 94.4% of patients, with a primary patency rate of 85.6% at more than three years. The limb salvage rate was 84.6% [36] (see **Figure 11**).

4. Conclusion

Both aortobifemoral bypass and endovascular aortoiliac reconstruction are effective and clinically efficient alternatives for the management of stenotic or occlusive aortoiliac disease. Recent contemporary literature reports comparable outcomes in patency, survival, and long-term limb preservation between the two techniques. The choice of procedure should be based on the clinical profile, age, surgical risk, and life expectancy of each patient to establish an effective long-term strategy. Further studies are needed to define the long-term durability of

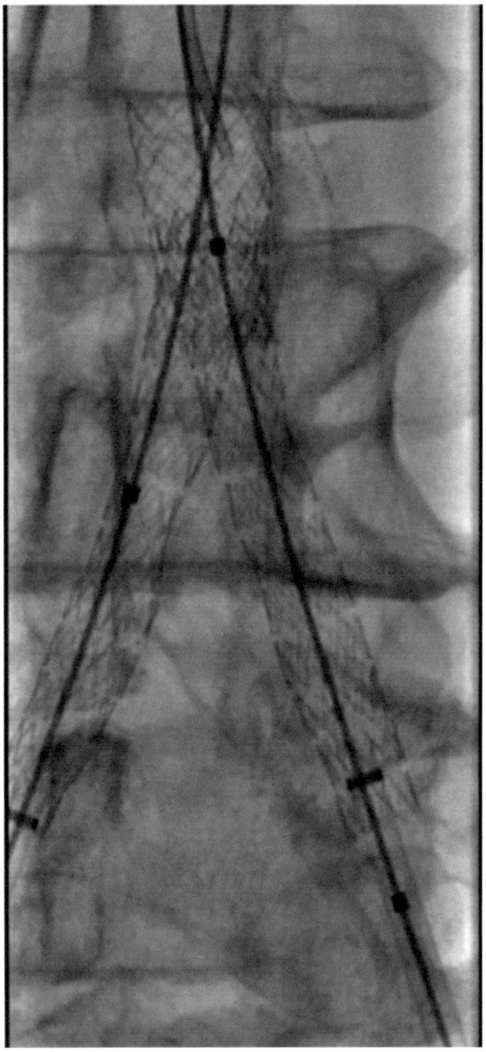

Figure 10.
Intraoperative radiograph demonstrating the stent configuration at the aortic bifurcation and correlation with the inferior mesenteric artery (IMA) stent. Tabiei et al. [37].

these endovascular approaches and to identify specific patient characteristics that may influence the outcomes of both endovascular approaches and open surgery.

Acknowledgments

Thanks to my wife Cristina, for her unconditional support, for always motivating me to pursue excellence, and for allowing me the space to express my ideas in projects like this. Thanks to my team: my assistant Miostys Melenciano, Dr. Mariel Cid (Surgeon), and Dr. Milvian Libarto (Anesthesiology), who share and facilitate great workdays filled with

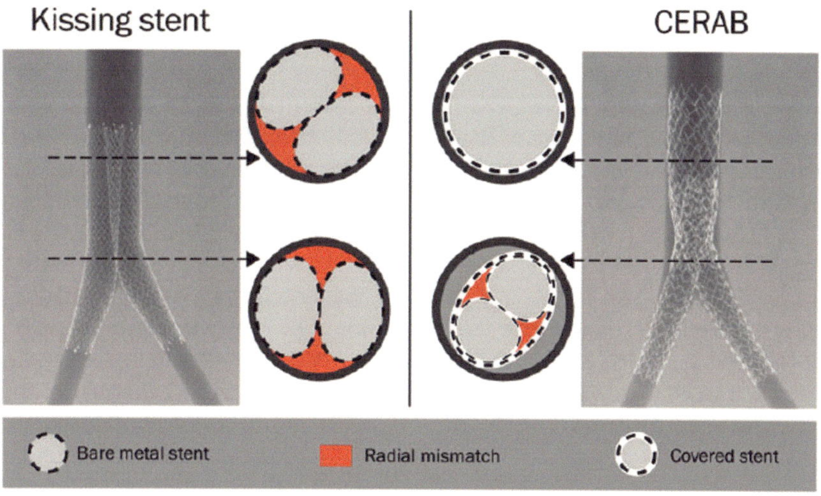

Figure 11.
Overview of the KS technique (left) using two self-expandable stents and the CERAB technique (right) using three balloon-expandable stents. For each configuration, two cross-sections are shown to depict the size of the in vitro *radial mismatch. CERAB: covered endovascular reconstruction of the aortic bifurcation; KS: kissing stent. Groot et al. [38].*

positive vibes and excellent results. Thanks to my colleagues and professors, with whom I discuss and share strategies and from whom I always receive recommendations based on the best experiences. Thanks to Unión Médica del Norte-CENICARDIO, for the optimal results on an extraordinary work platform.

Author details

Pedro Adolfo Mera Almonte
Medical Union, Santiago, Dominican Republic

*Address all correspondence to: pedroamera@gmail.com

References

[1] Leville CD, Kashyap VS, Clair DG, et al. Endovascular management of iliac artery occlusions: Extending treatment to TransAtlantic Inter-Society Consensus class C and D patients. Journal of Vascular Surgery. 2006;**43**:32–39

[2] Heaton J, Khan YS. Aortoiliac Occlusive Disease. NCBI Bookshelf. A Service of the National Library of Medicine. National Institutes of Health; 2020

[3] Gornik HL, Aronow HD, Goodney PP, Arya S, Brewster LP, Byrd L, Chandra V, Drachman DE, Eaves JM, Ehrman JK, Evans JN. 2024/ AHA/AACVPR/APMA/ABC/SCAI/ SVM/SVN/SVS/SIR/VESS guideline for the management of lower extremity peripheral artery disease: A report of the american college of cardiology/ american heart association joint committee on clinical practice guidelines. Circulation. 2024;**149**: e1313–e1410. DOI: 10.1161/ CIR.0000000000001251

[4] Desai S, Sharma D, Srinivas R, *et al.* Mesenchymal stromal cell therapy (REGENACIP®), a promising treatment option in chronic limb threatening ischemia – A narrative review. Stem Cell Research & Therapy. 2024;**15**:352

[5] Dave B, Shah R. Peripheral stent technology and current status for endovascular treatment of femoropopliteal artery disease: A clinical review. International Journal of Research in Medical Sciences. 2018;**6** (5):1474–1483. DOI: 10.18203/2320-601 2.ijrms20181743

[6] Mills JL, et al. The society for vascular surgery lower extremity threatened limb classification system: Risk stratification based on Wound, Ischemia, and foot Infection (WIfI). Journal of Vascular Surgery 2014;**59**:220–234.e2

[7] Bekken J, Vos JA, Aarts R, Vries JP, Fioole B. Discover: Dutch Iliac Stent trial: COVERed balloon-expandable versus uncovered balloon-expandable stents in the common iliac artery: Study protocol for a randomized controlled trial. Trials. 2012;**13:215**. DOI: 10.1186/ 1745–6215–13–215

[8] Norgren L, Hiatt WR, Dormandy JA, Nehler MR, Harris KA, Fowkes FG.Inter-society consensus for the management of peripheral arterial disease (TASC II). Journal of Vascular Surgery. 2007;**45**(1):S5–67

[9] Ogunsanya NL, Milner R, Delaney CL, Puckridge P. Aortoiliac occlusive disease – A novel classification system based on anatomical segments and disease severity for management planning. Vascular. 2024;**32**(5):1005–1014. DOI: 10.1177/17085381231166975

[10] ElSayed NA, Aleppo G, Aroda VR, Bannuru RR, Brown FM, Bruemmer D, et al. 6. glycemic targets: Standards of care in diabetes-2023. Diabetes Care 2023;**46**:S97–S110

[11] Weitz JI, Byrne J, Clagett GP, Farkouh ME, Porter JM, Sackett DL, et al. Diagnosis and treatment of chronic arterial insufficiency of the lower extremities: A critical review. Circulation. 1996;**94**(11)

[12] Gardner AW, Poehlman ET. Exercise rehabilitation programs for the treatment of claudication pain. A

meta-analysis. Jama. 1995;**274**(12):975–980

[13] Bouwens E, Klaphake S, Weststrate KJ, Teijink JA, Verhagen HJ, Hoeks SE, et al. Supervised exercise therapy and revascularization: Single-center experience of intermittent claudication management. Vascular Medicine 2019;**24**:208–215

[14] de Vries SO, Hunink MGM. Results of aortic bifurcation grafts for aortoiliac occlusive disease: A meta-analysis. Journal of Vascular Surgery. 1997;**26**:558–569

[15] Freyermuth M, Roisin S, Saidak Z, Matray L, Sevestre MA, Reix T, Soudet S. Contemporary minimally invasive surgery for TASC-D aorto-iliac lesions: Analysis of outcomes and risk factors for primary and secondary patency. Annals of Vascular Surgery. 2023;**97**:367–374. DOI: 10.1016/j.avsg.2023.05.018

[16] Hans SS, DeSantis D, Siddiqui R, Khoury M. Results of endovascular therapy and aortobifemoral grafting for Transatlantic Inter-Society type C and D aortoiliac occlusive disease. Surgery. 2008;**144**:583–589. Discussion 589–590

[17] Kashyap VS, Pavkov ML, Bena JF, Sarac TP, O'Hara PJ, Lyden SP, Clair DG. The management of severe aortoiliac occlusive disease: Endovascular therapy rivals open reconstruction. Journal of Vascular Surgery. 2008;**48**:1451–1457.1457e1451–1453

[18] Basílio-Martins M, Pereira-Neves A, Domingues-Monteiro D, Costa-Pereira T, Marques-Vieira M, Vidoedo J, Rocha-Neves J.Comparing endovascular and open reconstruction for TASC-II D aortoiliac disease: A propensity score analysis. International Surgery Journal. 2023;**11**(1):37–44

[19] Gao Z, Yue Y, Zhang Y, Jiang W, Zhang Y, Ran F, Li X. Comparison of clinical outcomes of endovascular therapy and hybrid surgery in the treatment of trans-atlantic inter-society consensus II D aortoiliac occlusive disease. International Journal of General Medicine. 2023;**16**:2149–2156. DOI: 10.2147/IJGM.S408609

[20] Chiu KW, Davies RS, Nightingale PG, Bradbury AW, Adam DJ.Review of direct anatomical open surgical management of atherosclerotic aorto-iliac occlusive disease. European Journal of Vascular and Endovascular Surgery. 2010;**39**(4):460–471

[21] Brown KN, Gonzalez L. StatPearls [Internet]. Leriche Syndrome(Archived). StatPearls Publishing: Treasure Island (FL); 2023.

[22] Dellehunt RE, Manna B Aortofemoral Bypass. Treasure Island (FL): StatPearls Publishing; 2025. Available from: https://www.ncbi.nlm.nih.gov/books/NBK542328/ [Accessed: 2023-Apr-19]

[23] Obitsu Y, Shigematsu H. Revascularization for the aortoiliac regions of peripheral arterial disease. Nihon Geka Gakkai Zasshi. 2010;**111**(2):79–83

[24] Bajardi G, Ricevuto G, Grassi N, Latteri M.Proximal anastomosis in aorto-bifemoral bypass. Technical considerations. Minerva Chirurgica. 1989;**44**(9):1353–1355

[25] Clair DG, Beach JM.Strategies for managing aortoiliac occlusions: Access, treatment and outcomes. Expert Review

of Cardiovascular Therapy. 2015;**13**(5):551–563

[26] Society for Vascular Surgery Lower Extremity Guidelines Writing Group, Conte MS, Pomposelli FB, et al. Society for Vascular Surgery practice guidelines for atherosclerotic occlusive disease of the lower extremities: Management of asymptomatic disease and claudication. Journal of Vascular Surgery. 2015;**61**(3 Suppl)

[27] Dikmen N, Ozcinar E, Akça F, Sen E, Karacuha AF, Kayan A, Yazicioglu L. The long-term results of covered endovascular aortic bifurcation repair in complex aortoiliac disease: A two-year follow-up. Journal of Clinical Medicine. 2024;**13**:5684. DOI: 10.3390/jcm13195684

[28] Dong X, Peng Z, Ren Y, *et al.* Tratamiento endovascular de la enfermedad oclusiva aortoilíaca con lesiones TASC II C y D: 10 años de experiencia en técnicas clínicas. BMC Cardiovascular Disorders. 2023;**23**(71). DOI: 10.1186/s12872-023-03059-4

[29] Gao Z, Yue Y, Zhang Y, Jiang W, Zhang Y, Ran F, Li X Comparison of clinical outcomes of endovascular therapy and hybrid surgery in the treatment of trans-atlantic inter-society consensus II D aortoiliac occlusive disease. International Journal of General Medicine. 2023;**16**:2149–2156. PMID: 37284037; PMCID: PMC10239638. DOI: 10.2147/IJGM.S408609

[30] Bekken JA, JA V, Aarts RA, de Vries JP, Fioole B DISCOVER: Dutch Iliac Stent trial: COVERed balloon-expandable versus uncovered balloon-expandable stents in the common iliac artery: Study protocol for a randomized controlled trial. Trials. 2012;**13**:215. DOI: 10.1186/1745-6215-13-215

[31] Bp M, Sharma S, Daneshmand A, SD T, et al. Durability of the balloon-expandable covered versus bare-metal stents in the Covered versus Balloon Expandable Stent Trial (COBEST) for the treatment of aortoiliac occlusive disease. Journal of Vascular Surgery 2016;**64**:83–94.e

[32] Zydlewski P, et al. Two-stage covered endovascular reconstruction of aortic bifurcation (CERAB) for patients with chronic limb-threatening ischemia. Journal of Vascular Surgery 2024;**79**:22

[33] Bontinis V, et al. Covered endovascular reconstruction of the aortic bifurcation: A systematic review aggregated data and individual participant data meta-analysis. Journal of Vascular Surgery 2024;**79**:1525–1535.e9

[34] Abdelbaqy OM, Holewijn S, Zeebregts CJ, Reijnen MM. The covered endovascular reconstruction of the aortic bifurcation (CERAB) technique for aorto-iliacocclusive disease. Surgical Technology Online. 2022;**40**:263–270. PMID: 35179733. DOI: 10.52198/22.STI.40.CV1542

[35] Pulli R, Dorigo W, Fargion A, Angiletta D, Azas L, Pratesi G, Innocenti AA, Pratesi C. Early and midterm results of kissing stent technique in the management of aortoiliac obstructive disease, annals of vascular surgery. Volume. 2015;**29**(3):543–550. DOI: 10.1016/j.avsg.2014.10.029

[36] Amanvermez Senarslan D, Yildırım F, Bayram B, Kurdal AT, Tetik O. Results of endovascular treatments of Trans-Atlantic Inter-Society Consensus C or D aortoiliac occlusive disease involving the aortic bifurcation. SAGE Open

Medicine. 2023;**11**:20503121231179836. PMID: 37674557; PMCID: PMC10478553. DOI: 10.1177/20503121231179836

[37] Tabiei A, Chait J, Cifuentes S, Haider A, Shuja F.Covered endovascular reconstruction of the aortic bifurcation with inferior mesenteric artery chimney for management of bilateral lower extremity tissue loss with concomitant mesenteric stenosis. Journal of Vascular Surgery Cases, Innovations and Techniques. 2023;**9**(2):101145

[38] Groot Jebbink E, Mors TG, Slump CH, Geelkerken RH, Holewijn S, Reijnen MM. In vivo geometry of the kissing stent and covered endovascular reconstruction of the aortic bifurcation configurations in aortoiliac occlusive disease. Vascular. 2017;**25**:635–641. DOI: 10.1177/1708538117708912